Extraordinary acclaim for

Melanoma: It Started With a Freckle

"At despair's doorstep, Dave Stanley gives us laughter, courage, and inspiration."

Dave Kindred, author of the Muhammad Ali/Howard Cosell dual biography Sound and Fury

David Stanley's story is human, factual and real. It shows the sunny road that seductively leads so many to cancer. Stanley uses his powerful story to present the facts and drama of melanoma. Best of all, he shows us how he comes through to the other side, a healthy, stronger person.

Fawn Germer, Oprah bestselling author with seven books on the New York Times *best-seller list and inspirational leadership speaker*

Men are far more likely than women to die of skin cancer. But as with other health issues that contribute to men's shorter, less-healthy lives, too many of us don't know enough about the risk factors, symptoms, and possible treatments. David Stanley eloquently and passionately weaves together his own personal story and the latest science, and has created a truly important book. Read it. It could save your life.

Armin Brott, Director of the top rated website, Talking About Men's Health, Time Magazine's *"Superdad's superdad" author and fatherhood expert*

The more melanoma awareness that is out there, the better. Melanoma can be a brutal disease. It's great that *Melanoma: It Started with a Freckle* will highlight the importance of skin checks and the need for advances in melanoma treatment.

Gillian Nuttall, founder of Melanoma UK

This short, readable, interesting book could save your life. I am probably alive today because years ago my wife nagged me into seeing a doctor about "moles" on my skin. Skin cancer is a huge public health problem, but a disease that is both preventable and—if caught early enough—treatable. Buy this book for someone you love.

David Hemenway, Ph.D., professor of Health Policy, Harvard School of Public Health, and director of the Harvard Injury Control Research Center and the Harvard Youth Violence Prevention Center

I imagine things for a living. When people read my work, I hope I'm sparking their imaginations. When I read another writer's book, I look forward to it sparking mine. So it sounds a little funny to say that one of the best things about *Melanoma: It Started with a Freckle* is that it doesn't leave me imagining a thing. I've never had cancer, and of course I don't want it. But if I ever do find myself in that situation, I now already know what I'm in for. I won't need the stress of having to imagine, and I won't have the unnecessary terror that comes with inevitably, naturally, and vividly imagining the worst possible version of every step. So thank you, David Stanley and only David Stanley, and just this once, for not letting me do what I do best. And for saving my life should I ever toss off a strange mole as no big deal. That I can imagine.

Jef Mallett, Award-winning cartoonist and creator of Frazz

This book, just possibly, might have saved MY life. I too spent decades in the sun on a bike and I too have a freckle. It might be nothing, but I would have ignored it accept for reading Dave's easily accessible, yet profound and data-driven memoir. Next week I have my second doctor's appointment in 34 years. Reading Dave's hijinks as a patient made me laugh, made me cry and made me continue to recognize that no matter our health, we all have a terminal illness called… LIFE. Time to "Really Live!"

John K. Coyle is an Olympic silver medalist in speedskating, NBC analyst, author, teacher, SVP, a professor of innovation

One of the biggest misconceptions about melanoma is that it is "just" skin cancer. David Stanley brilliantly illustrates that there's nothing "just" about it. On behalf of my father and many friends who fought the good fight against this disease but who are no longer with us, I thank David for penning such a powerful and candid description of his personal melanoma journey. His writings will warm the hearts of melanoma patients with similar experiences by letting them know they aren't alone and also will educate others to practice sun safety. Many thanks, David, for sharing your story so that others may learn and benefit from it.

Anita J. Day, Co-founder and Executive Director, Outrun the Sun, Inc., a nonprofit organization supporting skin cancer education and melanoma research: www.outrunthesun.org

David Stanley crafts a remarkable account of his journey with skin cancer. In the opening sentence of the Preface for *Melanoma: It Started with a Freckle*, Stanley sets a direct tone saying, "Everyone has a cancer story." Too many people do have cancer stories. Few writers craft the telling so well.

Without sentimentality and with wit, David's personal lens allows us to focus on the experience from the inside. For those of us with family members who have been affected by skin cancer, and for everyone who has yet to be affected, this is the book you want to read. And even a mention of Zingerman's as food heaven, his regular stop for post treatment meals, proves that Stanley know's what's important to say.

David Binder, this century's most esteemed photojournalist and the winner of the 2009 Athens Film festival for his film Calling My Children

In this book David Stanley wears his heart on his sleeve and bares his soul in order to get across the sickening disease that is melanoma. As a melanoma survivor myself, I can relate to every emotion that has overtaken David's life. Cancer doesn't just affect your health—it'll damage your whole life if you let it and the one thing you lose is control. Through David's honesty, integrity, humour and wit—*It Started with a Freckle* is a fascinating insight into one man's journey to fight, battle and survive melanoma. Being faced with death and not really knowing if you'll still be living to see your birthday, or Christmas—I can relate to David's change in attitude to the simple things in life. Every day is for living, for loving and appreciating the things we take for granted. Life is so precious, so are family and friends more than ever and it's been a privilege and a pleasure to share David's story. I send my very best wishes to him and his family for future good health.

Laura May McMullan, BBC journalist, and
Stage 3 melanoma survivor

David Stanley lets you know what it's like to be in his skin, literally. A riveting account of his experiences with melanoma is by turns suspenseful, affecting, and informative. Told with humor and intelligence, this book is a must read for anyone who wants to know more about the human side of this all-too-common cancer.

Lennard Davis, Ph.D., professor at the University of Illinois-Chicago, heard frequently on NPR, regarded as the leading U.S. voice on disability issues

David Stanley's memoir, *Melanoma: It Started with a Freckle*, is a must-read. By turns harrowing, insightful, technical, and hilarious, the book walks us through the frightening world of dealing with the deadliest form of skin cancer with humanity and humor. Stanley offers as much compassion for his care-givers as for his long-suffering family and brilliantly explains both the science and the emotional struggle involved in fighting cancer.

Tom Foster, Ph.D., author of How to Read Literature Like a Professor, *has had numerous appearances on the* New York Times *best-sellers list*

Dave Stanley's journey through melanoma will have you doing a double-take on your own skin. It will also equip you with life-saving information that could save your life—or the life of someone you love.

Jim Higley, award-winning author, cancer survivor, and TV personality

Melanoma

Melanoma

It Started with a Freckle

David L. Stanley

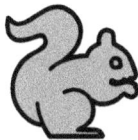

McGann Publishing
McMinnville, Oregon

Published by McGann Publishing
P.O. Box 864
McMinnville, OR 97128
USA
www.mcgannpublishing.com

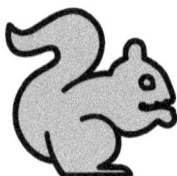

ISBN 978-0-9859636-6-8
Printed in the United States of America

For my wife, Cath, whose faith in me is unshakable.

For my parents, Mort and Lois, who urged me to find my own path.

And for my late brother Michael, who taught us all that "when going through Hell, keep going."

Acknowledgments

To the kind men and women who agreed to read a book by a new author and volunteered to put their acclaimed imprimaturs upon it with a blurb.

The men of the Dadbloggers group; men who work tirelessly, through their writing, to give a voice to fathers across the globe. Without the Saturday Night Drink thread, I'd have no reason to take photos of wine bottles, liquor, and odd makes of beer.

My colleagues at Dads Roundtable.com. Without their encouragement, and the platform that #DadsRT gave me, this book might not have seen the printed page.

A special thank-you to my #DadsRT colleague John "Hitchcock Tarantino" Willey and iCare Media for his peerless, selfless video work.

Mark Pelavin. He nudged me into doing a Jewish sports column for Reform Judaism.org's blog and here we are.

Nicole Zarins Tenenbaum. Her idea that "you know, those cancer stories of yours on your blog might make a pretty good book" proved to more prescient that either of us knew.

Larry Bernstein, of "Me, Myself, and Kids." A fine writer, his careful reading of the manuscript and subsequent suggestions were invaluable.

Prof. Tom Foster. The time I spent in study under Tom's tutelage created the voice that created this book. In addition, his reassurances always appeared at the proper moment.

Walter Barkey, MD, FAAD. His careful exams saved my life. His careful writing created a darn fine foreword.

Blue. Miles Davis and *Kind of Blue*. Oatmeal with butter, brown sugar, and blueberries. Gershwin's *Rhapsody in Blue*. Dylan's *Tangled up in Blue*. Always there when I needed them.

Aunt Susan Bramson. Outside of a dog, a book is man's best friend. Inside of a dog it's too dark to read.

Kerry, BP, and Amy Jo. My beige pod buddies, colleagues, and cheer-
leaders.

Joan Ring. My high school English teacher who taught me the meaning of the word parsimony and how best to achieve it.

E.B. White. "Omit needless words." Yes, sir.

Bill McGann, a man who was willing to take a chance on my work.

Carol McGann, patient and wise: un editor senza uguali.

My son Aaron, for his persistent piercing of my balloon.

My parents, Mort and Lois, who encouraged a guy to head down every
path that caught his eye.

My late brother Michael, who gave me resolve when I wavered, in life
and death.

Cathy, my wife. This book is for her.

Contents

Part Five: The Encore, and Meet and Greet in the Lobby

Appendices

About the Author

Foreword

Although we may prefer not to think about it much, no one needs to be told that we are all going to die of something eventually. Cardiovascular disease (i.e., strokes and heart attacks) and cancer are the big killers in the industrialized world. In the last 30 years there have been tremendous advances in the prevention and treatment of cardiovascular disease. These advances have had a significant impact on our longevity. One unfortunate side effect of this improved cardiovascular survival is that when people live longer, they are more likely to succumb to cancer of one form or another. Although everyone knows that life is finite and that no one has yet discovered the secret to immortality, being diagnosed with cancer is like a slap in the face that makes you suddenly have to face your own mortality.

For me growing up, cancer was some obscure entity that affected mostly old people I didn't know that I assumed were going to die of something anyway. Then, when you or someone close to you is diagnosed with cancer, it really puts a face on it. David Stanley's *Melanoma: It Started with a Freckle* certainly does that. Once the diagnosis of cancer is made, each doctor visit, each procedure, each setback, is another act in this ultra-personal true life drama, this "battle" between you, and in David's case, that "rat bastard melanoma." David's perspective is colored by his scientific roots and his desire as a teacher to inform his audience. But it is his humor and wit that really bring the message home and make it real.

As David points out, melanoma is a killer, but unlike almost any other cancer, the death rate from melanoma has been actually increasing over the past four decades. This has been despite well publicized efforts to educate the public about melanoma recognition including the introduction of the ABCDs of melanoma recognition in the mid-1980s. As a dermatologist in training 35 years ago I felt that dying of a melanoma that was staring you right in the face just asking to be found at a curable stage seemed so unnecessary and the remedy seemed very obvious. Since melanoma is right out there where anyone can see it, why don't we just teach everyone what it looks like and then remove them all at an early curable stage? After all, no one wants to die of something "stupid" they should have been paying attention to.

The trouble is that many melanomas are not detected with the ABCDs, there are millions of us that have ABCD lesions that are totally benign, and there are access problems to good dermatologic care.

Over the past 35 years of practice working with real people who get real melanomas, I've tried to come up with some answers. In dermatology, there isn't nearly enough manpower to screen every person every year so there has to be some priority given to high risk people who are the ones most likely to develop melanoma. Melanomas mostly come from sun you get in the first 30 years of your life and therefore any preventative measures should be directed at very young people (and their parents) regarding sun protection (e.g., sunscreens and protective clothing) and avoidance of tanning spas. So seeing people after age 30 it's more about early detection than prevention.

Although melanomas do occur in African Americans and people who tan very easily ("olive" or "Mediterranean" skin types), it primarily affects those with Fitzpatrick Skin Types I (burns easily and never tans) and II (usually burns first and then tans). I don't mind teaching anyone that is interested about melanoma recognition but everyone with Skin Types I and II should all be taught how a melanoma may look or act at a stage when it can be cured, just as people who live in wooden buildings should be taught fire drills that they should practice on a regular basis. You still might die in a fire anyway but you stand a better chance of surviving if you practiced a drill.

The following is what I try to teach people every day in my office who I am screening for melanoma and who want to be empowered with potential life-saving information about its early recognition.

First, there are only two things a melanoma can arise from, real moles and normal skin. There are all kinds of harmless things we grow later in life and learning how to recognize these and to distinguish them from melanoma is an important life skill. You don't want to waste any time and energy looking at hereditary scaly growths, skin tags, red "cherry" angiomas, and the like as they have no malignant potential whatsoever. When I see a patient for a skin cancer screen I examine every inch of their body. While I do this, I educate them about melanoma recognition and I try to point out their "real moles" that have at least some cancer risk. These are usually flat freckle-like brown moles that have been present since early childhood, as about 20% of melanomas come from this type of mole. Although roughly only about 1 in 10,000 of these moles per year turns into a melanoma, these are the only type of mole you really need to "keep an eye on." With these real moles we only care about a new asymmetric change. Since many of these are located on the back or other less visible sites, a partner is needed to help monitor these.

The other 80% of melanomas are a new spot that arises in previously normal looking skin. So how are these recognized and separated from the dozens of benign things we all grow with age? I like to instruct patients using a baseball analogy. You are up to bat and of course, trying not to strike out. "New" is one strike. Since the vast majority of melanomas arise *de novo* (i.e., just pop up where there was nothing), anything new must get close attention. You don't strike out with one strike but you look at the next few pitches more closely when you already have one strike against you. A possible second strike would be, "doesn't match my other growths." This is known as the "ugly duckling sign." The opposite of this is when you already have three or four similar growths and this new one looks just like them. Melanomas don't come in pairs or triplets. Melanoma is the lone wolf, the "ugly duckling."

Another possible strike would be "flat and brown." Most early melanomas are flat and brown (like David's "Freckle") and this alone wouldn't let you distinguish an age spot from a melanoma. But with age spots there should be no "ugly duckling sign." Several other potential big time strikes would be "has some irregularity of color and/or border" and "just seems to keep growing continuously over time." Melanomas are cancer and they grow at different rates. But even the slowest growing ones change over time (i.e., month to month).

For those individuals who make hereditary brown scaly growths called seborrheic keratoses, I try to help them recognize that melanomas do not typically make any true scale and that any growth in such people that is clearly scaly is like getting hit by a pitch when up to bat, a free pass to first base.

I then like to tell people that their job isn't to figure out if something is actually a melanoma, their job is just to screen for things that have two or more strikes and *might* be a melanoma. My job as a dermatologist isn't to actually just look at something and tell whether it is a melanoma or not either. There are a lot of benign things that I can positively identify by their appearance (both to the visible eye and on dermoscopy) and palpable features. But if a new growth is not clearly one of these benign lesions then my job is also to determine if one of these *might* be a melanoma and to biopsy any such thing and have it read by a competent dermatopathologist.

High risk people (people with Skin Types I and II, people who have a family history of melanoma in a parent or sibling, people who frequented tanning spas more than 100 times before age 25, people who spent lots of time outdoors growing up and had some severe blistering sunburns, and people with lots of larger moles) should establish a relationship with a melanoma expert (usually a dermatologist) and be shown which lesions they have that need monitoring. This expert should be someone who can see you on a timely basis (e.g. less than a month) if you develop a new suspicious lesion. What good is an expert if you don't have timely access?

It's easy to say that you should see such an expert once a year for screening. There are simply not enough dermatologists out there to do this. I practice in a county with over 450,000 people and there are 5 dermatologists. Even if I did 50 screenings five days a week I could only see 12,500 people a year. Even with three competent PAs that work side by side with me we couldn't screen all these people. And if I tried and someone tried to call me urgently with a new suspicious lesion, I wouldn't be able to accommodate him or her. I'd be too busy doing screenings. The average wait time to see a dermatologist is three months in most areas of the country.

Therefore, I think it is best to establish a relationship with a dermatologist, learn what needs monitoring and what does not and learn in person and with pictures the warning signs (i.e., "strikes") of early melanomas. Then this graduate of "Melanoma 101" needs to be able to contact this expert and have a timely screening for anything with two or more strikes. Yearly screening is inefficient and impractical and adds to the wait time of people who have new concerning lesions that need to be evaluated on a timely basis. My staff has been carefully taught to screen calls to figure out if someone (or some referring doctor's office) is calling because they are concerned about a new or changing growth that might be malignant. These people are told at the time of their first screening to be "the squeaky wheel" when they call if they are concerned about malignancy.

But even if medical providers such as myself are able to come up with more practical and effective strategies to find more melanomas at an early treatable stage, how do we get people to start paying attention like it could really happen to them? Without awareness there is no chance of motivating people to look at their own skin with a critical eye for new and/or suspicious lesions that might actually be vitally important.

David's intensely personal story and his unique perspective as a teacher and scientist certainly go a long way towards making melanoma "real" to readers. David also has a unique ability to entertain as he "lets us into his head" during his fascinating medical saga filled with humor and pathos.

Walter Barkey, MD, FAAD
Flint, Michigan
November, 2015

Preface
Why Melanoma? Why Now?

Everyone has a cancer story. Cancer strikes fathers and mothers, brothers and sisters, children, nieces and nephews, loved ones and trusted friends, and everyone in between. Over the course of a lifetime, 40% of us will develop a cancer of some kind. Half of those attacked by cancer will die.

So why is this story, a melanoma story, in particular, important? Because melanoma is the only cancer, of the seven most common cancers, in which the incidence continues to grow. Since 2000, melanoma diagnoses have increased 2% every year. One out of fifty adults will develop melanoma during their lifetime. The incidence of squamous cell skin carcinomas has increased: doubled since the mid-1980s. Over the past thirty years, more people have had skin cancer than all other cancers combined. So, why don't we do more to protect ourselves?

Skin cancer in general, and melanoma in particular, suffers from a lack of awareness and press. It is not possible to watch television for more than an hour without seeing an anti-smoking commercial. Over the course of my lifetime, those commercials have, rightfully, become stark and graphic. As the pool of smokers shrinks, it takes more and more to budge those few smokers who remain to put down their Winstons.

But skin cancers face a tougher battle. Tanned skin looks good. Pale skin looks pasty, sallow, wan, ashen. According to an IBIS World report, the tanning industry has grown just over 3% annually since 2000, and generates about $5 billion dollars in revenue. That's a lot of money for a product that when used regularly, is more effective than tobacco at causing cancer. Indeed, the Skin Cancer Foundation has found that more people develop skin cancer because of indoor tanning than there are smokers who develop lung cancer from smoking. The World Health Organization includes indoor tanning machines in its Group 1 carcinogens: the most dangerous cancer-causing agents. Group 1 also includes plutonium and cigarettes.

David L. Stanley

It's not just the fashionistas among us. We like to get outside. Here in southeast Michigan, the summer exodus via I-75 to our local vacation land, the northern half of Michigan's Lower Peninsula, begins every Friday around noon. The freeway begins to fill up with cars and trucks and RVs and campers and boats. By early evening, northbound I-75 resembles Daytona Speedway. The Friday exodus from mid-town Manhattan to the Hamptons is no different. The weekend traffic from Philadelphia to Avalon, New Jersey is so dense that it might well be possible to walk the 80 miles faster, from hood to hood of the barely moving cars, than to drive.

What's on everybody's agenda? Getting outside and getting some sun. We crave sunshine. In small doses, or protected with proper sunscreen, that sun soothes the soul, and makes the work week tolerable.

We conveniently ignore this statistic: five sunburns as a youth double your chances of developing melanoma as an adult. That's not five in a year. That's five. Full stop. That's all it takes to permanently degrade your DNA over the course of your life. Once you've had melanoma, you are nine times more likely than the general population to develop another one.

The economic costs are also significant. The US loses about $3 billion in productivity every year due to melanoma. We spend $8 billion every year in skin cancer treatment. The average annual treatment cost increase for other cancers, since 2001, has been around 25% every year. For skin cancers, that annual increase is 125%.

I was lucky. My cancer was spotted early. When my melanoma came back, my care team was able to excise my cancer with minimal disfigurement. Many of the people I met in waiting rooms were not so lucky. I met people who were missing salad plate sized pieces of scalp. I met a woman without a nose. I saw several people who had an external ear removed. One lost an ear and the tissue surrounding that ear and much of the tissue around that side's eye. I met a man who had an eye removed due to melanoma of the eye. These men and women, like all cancer warriors, ran the gamut. Stoic, tranquil, petrified, garrulous, resigned; over the course of my treatment, I was all of these, and so were these people.

Skin cancers exist in a blurred world. It starts with dermatology. Part of the skin cancer world is oncology. Part of the world is plastic and reconstructive surgery. Yet, for many skin cancer patients, their world may end with brain surgery.

My melanoma started with a freckle. But the cure started with dermatology.

Dermatology: it's not just zits and Botox anymore.

Part One
The Prelude

The First Freckle

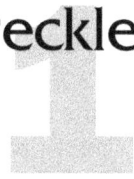

1

"This is the face of cancer," I thought as my virtual image stared back at me from my bathroom mirror. I looked in my eyes. When I gazed at the right side of my face, I could see laugh lines around my blue eyes. My forehead was relaxed. Wrinkly, as befits a fifty-year-old man, but relaxed. I could watch my breath ruffle my nostrils and fog the mirror as I worked my shaving brush around my nose. The right side of my face looked fine. It was shaved. It was clean. It was… *my face*.

But the left side; that was not my face. The left side of my face was a patchwork quilt woven by a surgeon's exquisite touch. I turned my head so I could see my face's left side and studied the image in the mirror. Terror and disgust stared back at me. I wanted to smash the mirror. I wanted to form a fist and drive it through the looking glass, through the drywall, and out the other side, cuts and broken knuckles be damned.

The left side of that face—*that* side of my face now belonged to a monster; a monster that would take over its host's body and quite willingly rot it out from the inside. A monster called melanoma.

Melanoma starts out easily enough. A small clump of your skin's pigment cells break free from their genetic on/off switches. Much like an anthill, little goes on that can be seen from the surface. Yet, below the skin's upper boundary, your wayward melanocytes are busy as they tunnel about below the surface. A tumor five millimeters across may harbor dozens of tunnels, each ten times longer than the tumor, as the tumor readies itself to spread throughout your body.

My first glimpse at the face of cancer barely rattled me. A needle stick and a surgical scrape, followed a short time later by another needle stick and a snip of skin, plus two stitches and a band-aid. Easy. Painless. Done.

My second glimpse at the face of cancer brought the terror of cancer home like a leather-masked man with a chainsaw in a grindhouse movie. This cancer was back and it was angry.

This cancer brought its own set of biopsies. From the first biopsy, there were red and blue tattoo scars. There were forty small, neatly tied sutures, in a square one and one-quarter inches directly in front of my ear.

From the second biopsy, there was another larger square which emanated out from that first square in an odd optical illusion. There were sixty more stitches, still small and neatly tied, marking the territory like a firebreak. More tattoo dye, still alternating red and blue, underlay the needlework.

The third biopsy drew another line further out around the original lesion. This limit was nearly as long as any two of the other tattooed lines combined.

I was unable to shave around the operative site. Grizzled hair sprouted at odd angles in, around, and over the nested squares. That face resembled a farmer's cutover corn field in October: the remnants of cut down corn stalks, nibbled and shredded by deer and raccoon, bewhiskered and dead brown.

That face. That face was not my own. That face belonged to melanoma and I was driven to reclaim it as my own.

My melanoma started with a freckle. I had a freckle on the left side of my face. I couldn't see it. My wife, my lovely Cath, R.N., B.S.N, M.S.N. noticed it one September evening in 2005.

"You got a weird thing on your face," she said.

"Huh? Weird how? Like food? A dead moth? Dandruff? Where?" I answered.

She leaned over and touched my cheek, an inch in front of my tragus: the nubbin of flesh in front of the ear canal.

"Right there. It's kind of brown and grey."

"So? Big deal. I got a thing. I get sun splotches all the time. Zits. Whatever."

I shrugged.

Cath put on her reading glasses and gave it a good going-over. She had me turn towards the light. She tugged on my tragus. She looked at from different angles. She grabbed the skin near my sideburn and stretched out the area just in front of my ear.

"This is different. It's not right. You need to get it looked at."

I made my "yeah, right, whatever" face. I waved my hand at her.

She wasn't kidding.

"Don't look at me like that. I'm being a health care provider here."

I recognized her tone. I recognized her look. She had put on her nurse's hat. I made an appointment with the family dermatologist.

"Flint Dermatology, Dr. Barkey's office. How may I help you?"

Melanoma: It Started With a Freckle

"Um, yeah, my wife is a nurse and she says I have this weird freckle in front of my ear that needs to be looked at."

"Yes. We just had a cancellation. Doctor can see you Tuesday at 4:00 pm next week. Or we're booking six weeks from now."

Tuesday, at 4 pm, I found myself sitting in an exam chair. Dr. Walter Barkey, MD, FAAD, a board certified dermatologist, was breathing into my ear as he looked at my "weird freckle" through a highly technical magnifying glass.

Barkey is a University of Michigan man, right down to the ground. Phi Beta Kappa, B.A, M.D., all earned in Ann Arbor. He has U-M gear stylishly arranged in his waiting room, and quite possibly, a Block-M bumper sticker on his Audi TT in the parking lot.

He is also exceedingly bright, pleasant, and he diagnosed my mother's rare dermatological condition of pemphigus when no other physician was able. I trust him.

"Hmm, yes. Hmm, David, we need a biopsy for that. It'll take a moment. I have several concerns about this. It *is* something. I don't want to alarm you with that. It's small. We're early. I am concerned, but there's no need to be scared. But it is certainly a something. The question is what sort of something? Here, I'll show you."

I heard a camera whrr. Dr. Barkey handed me the camera. It was my freckle, blown up ten times.

"Take a look."

He pointed to the sawtooth edges of my freckle with a pen.

"See how the edges are erose, kind of jagged? That's often a sign that it's some sort of skin cancer."

Dr. Barkey pointed back and forth on the freckle; from the brown to the grey and back again.

"See how it is several different colors? That's not good, either.

"Right off the bat, this *something* of yours has two of skin cancer's warning signs. Again, and I really feel the need to repeat this, is not a big deal. This should be very manageable. But first, before I can draw any conclusions, we need a biopsy. No guesswork allowed. Just the data.

"Let's talk about the biopsy for a moment, okay? You've had stitches and all that before, yes? Well, the biopsy is no big deal, then, compared to getting a cut stitched up in ER. It's simple. I'll numb it up, just a little Novocain, and I'll use this little melon baller to take a tissue sample."

He held up what looked like a dental tool with a sesame seed sized scoop on the end.

"I may put in a stitch, just to be sure, and send off your sample to the path lab. We'll know something by the end of the week."

I nodded in agreement.

"Sounds good. You're in charge, Walt. I trust you. We do this right now, or do I need to come back later?"

"You're here, I've got the time, let's do this now, if that works for you," he said.

"Showtime, then," I said.

"I'm going to go see a patient in the next room, Dave, while you get prepped. You lay down on your side, I'll have my assistant put a drape over the side of your face, clean you up a bit, and then I'll be back. Should take about five minutes for your prep, and maybe less for the biopsy. I've done a lot of these; I kind of have it down."

He smiled, a broad and confident smile.

"Good?"

I nodded again.

"Good," I said.

Dr. Barkey's assistant took command. She was every bit as pleasant as the chief.

"Okay, need you to swing your legs around, so you're sitting cross-ways on the chair…"

I swung around 90 degrees.

"Perfect," she said. "Now, I'm going to lean the chair back, so you're going to go over sideways. Here's a pillow. Just go along for the ride, that's the easiest way."

The chair hummed. I tipped over on my side like a Weeble.

The assistant tore open a swab from a foil packet and gently swiped and daubed the side of my face. It had a cooling effect.

"Okay, now for the drape."

From a surgical kit, she produced a piece of blue-grey hospital paper about one foot on each edge. It had a hole about two inches square in its center. She covered the left side of my face; my ear, up to my hair-line, down to my jawline. Twisting my eyes in their sockets up towards the ceiling, I could see the outline of the bright examination room light through the paper. The drape had looked rough as she shook it open, but felt smooth on my face.

I could hear her bustle around—a clink of glass on metal as she placed the small bottle of local anesthetic on a tray, a tearing sound as she opened the biopsy kit.

I heard three footsteps and, in the hall, a muffled woman's voice: "Dr. Barkey? We're ready when you are."

As I lay there, I could hear bits of Dr. Barkey's conversation with his other patient. I could hear flesh meet flesh as he shook hands with his patient. I could hear the swoosh of his lab coat against his street clothes as he turned and walked into my room. Odd, the things you can hear when you are lying on your side, face covered in a surgical drape, and all you can see is the wall directly opposite your face.

As Dr. Barkey walked into the room, he spoke. I could hear rubber slap as he put on his gloves.

"Okay, Dave. Here's what's going to happen. I have a skinny little derm needle here. I'll numb you up, wait a few seconds for the local to take effect, and then I'll do the biopsy. I'm taking such a small amount of tissue; you might not even feel any pressure. Maybe a stitch, I'll see once I do the biopsy, but probably just a steri-strip. Good? Any questions? Can we get started?"

"Just one. How skinny is that needle? Just curious, I've had like a hundred, hundred and fifty stitches."

"Skinny. Like acupuncture needles. You can hardly feel it."

I felt the weight of his hand on the side of my face. His hand rested partly on my ear.

"Here goes," he said. "Feel that?"

"Not even."

"Little burn now."

It felt like an unhappy mosquito.

"Okay, time for the biopsy. Don't move for a moment."

I heard a brief sound that reminded me of a slice of bread as it was cut from a loaf.

"There. And we're done."

He turned to his assistant, "Steri-strip is fine.

"Want to see?"

He held a small glass container in front of my still horizontal face. A piece of my face the size and color of a sesame seed floated in the liquid. His assistant removed the drape, the chair hummed, and I was gently returned to an upright position.

"This will go off to the lab today. I do believe that you have skin cancer, but I promise, this will be easily manageable. It's early and it's very small. So, please, no lost sleep. Business as usual. I'll call you late Thursday afternoon and we'll discuss your results."

It's Cancer: Specifically, It's Melanoma

My phone rang late Thursday afternoon.

"Dave? Walt Barkey here. I have your results back. No surprise, you have skin cancer. More specifically, you have melanoma. You might know that melanoma is potentially, hear me now, just potentially in your case, the most dangerous kind of skin cancer. But, of all possible melanoma cases, yours is the best. It's what we call *in situ*. That means that the tumor is still confined to its original location. In the case of melanoma, that means it hasn't yet sent out any little runners under your skin. This is a good case scenario. Melanoma can be sneaky. That's how it spreads."

"So it's encysted?" I asked.

Some micro-organisms can grow cysts, a hard shell-like casing, around themselves when conditions get tough. It's a great evolutionary trick to survive highly dangerous environments. I'm a high school science teacher by profession but by degree, I'm a zoologist with a histochemistry minor thrown in the mix. I understand the science of this. My father is a physician. My wife is a nurse. I worked as an emergency room orderly as an undergrad. I know the words, and I know what they mean.

"Not exactly, but you're close." he said, laughing. "You speak the language. Okay."

"Your tumor is *in situ*. *In situ* means 'in site' or 'in location.' That's how early we caught it. It hasn't started to spread and that's perfect. So, while it's not enclosed, it is all in one piece. Kind of like a chocolate chip that hasn't started to melt.

"You do need to have it removed as soon as possible, but if there is a best way to have melanoma, *in situ* is the best way. I don't do these cases. I'll have my staff call Dr. Alghanem, he's my usual guy for cases like this, if that's okay. He's a plastic surgeon and he does a lot of skin cancer work. Unless you have someone else you'd like to use?"

"No, that's fine," I said. "If he's the guy you like to use, like I said, I trust your judgment. I sort of know him. Our kids play on an AYSO soccer team I coach. Seems like a good guy. Should I block out the day, or is this a no big deal office procedure? Will I be able to go back to work the next day?"

"At this stage, it's no big deal," said Dr. Barkey. "He'll do it in the office, local anesthesia, a couple stitches to seal the deal, ice pack in the evening, back to work the next day. I'm going to hand the phone over to our scheduler. She'll take care of you. I want to see you two weeks after he does your face. Oh, and make sure you thank your wife, because she's the one who caught this so early. You're lucky. This is an easy one."

Four days later, on Monday afternoon, I found myself sitting in Dr. Abd Alghanem's office; draped, numb and nervous. That I had assurances about my case from a doctor I trusted didn't help. That the surgeon was well thought of by both my doctor and several of my doctor-friends didn't help. That this was an outpatient procedure didn't help. That I'd be heading straight to practice with the Holly High School soccer team I also coach after the procedure didn't help.

I had cancer. Not just your everyday basal cell carcinoma: the skin cancer of lifeguards and lawn-mowing guys. Basal cell is so common that if you live to 65, the odds are 50/50 that you'll develop a basal cell skin cancer. Three million people per year in the USA are diagnosed with basal cell carcinoma. It can disfigure, but it rarely kills.

No, I had melanoma. The cancer that took down Bob Marley. And TV producer icon Stephen Cannell of the Rockford Files. And Bruce Springsteen's keyboard player Danny Federici. President Reagan's daughter Maureen died of melanoma at age 62. In my case, caught in time, easy enough to manage, but nonetheless, melanoma.

My surgery was no more draining than the biopsy. I lay on my side. Dr. Alghanem chatted in my ear about our school age boys on the soccer field. His melon baller was bigger than Barkey's. The doctor wore magnifying glasses over his regular glasses. The incision was ¾ of an inch long. He showed me his work in a mirror. He was calm. I could hear his deep, regular breathing. As I managed my low-grade anxiety, I counted my breaths.

One, two, three, four. One, two, three, four. I could hear my heartbeat in my right ear, the ear pressed against the seat cushion of Alghanem's exam room chair.

"Just a normal day at the office," I told myself.

I felt a little pressure as he pulled the sutures through my skin. More clearly, I heard it as he pulled the sutures through my skin. Dr.

Alghanem put in several stitches, not much bigger than thick hairs, to add to my lifetime count. Fifteen minutes start to finish, he was done, and I was bandaged. He snapped off his gloves, and we shook hands.

"Make sure you schedule your follow-up appointment for next Thursday on your way out," said Dr. Alghanem. "We'll take out your stitches. This procedure went very well. You'll be fine with an icepack and Tylenol. If it hurts more than that, call me please. I need to know about it.

"See you Saturday at the kids' soccer game."

I was done. We shook hands and I was out the door, into my tan GMC Safari minivan and off to soccer practice. No pain.

I arrived at high school soccer practice a few minutes late. I had told my assistant coach that I'd be late, and he was welcome to tell the team.

"Hey, coach! How'd it go?" I heard as I walked onto the field.

I showed them the silver dollar size bandage on the left side of my face, directly in front of my ear. I told them I had melanoma, most likely due to all the time I spent in the sun whilst I was playing soccer and racing bicycles from my teens to my early thirties. I urged them all to wear sunscreen. We went back to practice.

Several hours later, after dinner with my wife and my thirteen year old son shaggy headed tennis playing son Aaron, I peeled back the band-aid.

Cath peered at the surgical site. For several years, she worked in a branch of a hospital where plastic surgery was commonplace. She tipped my head from side to side to get the best light.

She tipped her head from side to side. She slid her reading glasses up and back on her nose.

"He did nice work. Very clean lines. Very neat knots," she said.

"Good to know," I responded.

"Aaron, I had a little bit of surgery today."

"Yeah, I see that," he said. "What's up?"

"I had a skin cancer removed. Not a big deal. Dr. Alghanem did it right in the office. A little shot, a couple of nicks with the scalpel, the two stitches you see. I'm good to go."

"Dr. Alghanem? Fares' dad?"

"Yessir."

I could see his mind as he put his soccer teammate's dad into scrubs and gloves at the office.

"Skin cancer?"

"Yessir."

"A little skin cancer?" he asked.

"Yessir," I said.

"They got it all? No cancer left behind? It won't come back?"

"Well, they said they got it all. They also said it could come back, but they said I'm no more likely to have it come back than any other random guy who spent too much time in the sun."

"So, it's all good?"

"As far as I know."

"I shouldn't worry, then?"

"No. No worries."

"Okay, then I won't."

"Good choice."

Twenty months later, on a Monday in May, 2007, Cath and I were talking at the dinner table. She stopped in mid-sentence and leaned in close. I thought she wanted to kiss. I was good with that. She was not interested in kissing. She was staring at the side of my face. The left side of my face, directly in front of my tragus.

"Your thing is back," she stated.

"Wha? My thing?"

"Your freckle."

She touched a spot directly in front of my ear.

"It's back. Bigger, too. Lots. Maybe one and a half centimeters across. It's right on the suture line from the old one."

"You're not kidding, are you?" I said. "How much bigger?"

"I'd never kid about something like this. Twice as big, easy. In both directions."

"Jagged-like?" I asked.

"On one side. And it's a couple different shades of gray and brown."

"Shit," I said. "This can't be good."

The Mean Streets of Melanoma

That I should have skin cancer did not surprise me. Born in 1958, sunscreen was only used the first few days of the summer to lay down a "base tan". The base tan was a mythical beast that gave us "protection" against sun damage throughout the summer. In his cartoon *Doonesbury*, Gary Trudeau spoofed the 1970s tan craze with his character Zonker, a professional stoner/tanner who won the George Hamilton Pro-Am Celebrity Cocoa Butter Open. During the mid-1970s, we often used coconut oils as tanning accelerants. Tans looked good. Tans felt good. A fact ignored by college students of that era, tans also created permanent skin damage and alterations to our skin's DNA.

I did not always tan well. I was always a "burn first, tan later" guy. My family roots are from the Ukraine and Lithuania. We are a fair-skinned, northern hemispheric people. Those of us with roots at the Earth's 50th parallel did not have much evolutionary need for high levels of melanin as did my Greek friends from the 35th parallel.

My athletic habits did not help. I was a soccer player through high school and college, out in the sun all day long, often shirtless, all summer long. My summer jobs as a youth soccer coach and lawn mower exposed me to even more sun. Unknown to me at the time, sun damage is cumulative. My youth would catch up with me.

Heck, I tanned. I loved to lay in the sun at the Michigan State outdoor pool when I was in college. There were girls there. Girls who loved to lay out. Very attractive girls in very small swimsuits basking in the sun on a college campus. What college guy would not want to be there?

I even competed in the Charles "Lash" Larrowe Cocoa-butter Classic whilst at Michigan State. Larrowe was an MSU economics professor who enjoyed hanging out at the pool whilst ogling the bikini-clad MSU coeds. What's a hottie-loving prof to do in the summer? Start a tanning contest.

It gets worse. For most of my twenties, I was an itinerant semi-pro bicycle racer. I was on a bike from three to six hours every day, nine months a year. Early season training was done in Florida and Austin, Texas. Latitude 30° South.

Sunscreen? We don't need no stinkin' sunscreen.

Melanoma can be a very efficient killer. Nearly 9,000 people were killed by melanoma in 2012. Over 80,000 new US-based cases of melanoma were reported in 2012. Rates of new cases have doubled since 1980. Depending on your race, gender, and geographic location, melanoma may be as high as number four with a literal bullet on your cancer hit parade. It is on the Top Ten list of cancer killers, regardless of other factors. Melanoma accounts for only 5% of all skin cancer diagnoses, yet it accounts for 75% of all skin cancer deaths. It's not good to have melanoma. Reggae icon Bob Marley died in 1981. His melanoma started under a toenail.

Why is melanoma, cancer of the body's pigment cells, the melanocytes, so deadly? One, melanocytes are common throughout the body. Where are melanocytes found? Wherever you have color: the skin, the middle layer of the eye (the uvea), the inner ear, meninges, bones, the heart, you have melanocytes.

Two, melanoma is a sneaky bastard. Melanoma can grow down into your skin from a Rice Krispy sized lesion on the surface and race out many centimeters under your skin. Melanoma can camouflage itself from your body's immune system. Deadliest of all, melanoma likes to, in the words of Dr. Barkey, "go home to the brain."

As embryos, humans have three basic germ layers. Those basic tissue layers are the endoderm, mesoderm, and ectoderm. Every cell in your body can trace its development back to one of these three germ cell types. You may recall from Bio 9 in high school that skin is derived from ectoderm. Melanocytes, the skin's pigment cells, are also derived from ectoderm. Our brains, too, are also derived from ectoderm. Brain cells and melanocytes are produced from neural crest cells, both of which are derived from ectoderm. All of these cells derived from ectoderm, when melanoma strikes, show a marked affinity for each other.

For reasons not well understood, melanoma lesions like to go in search of their relatives. In other words, the cancerous melanocytes want to take up residence in your brain. Melanoma, unchecked, often travels to your brain and causes brain metastases. Quite simplistically, melanoma can cause brain tumors. That's what killed Bob Marley—the brain tumors. At this writing in the summer of 2015, it has just been announced that President Jimmy Carter has brain lesions as a result of his melanoma.

Melanoma: It Started With a Freckle

Our skin is comprised of three main layers: the outer epidermis, the middle dermis, and the lower level, the hypodermis. Sunlight is made up of a wide spectrum of light frequencies. Ultraviolet (UV) light, comprised of UVA and UVB frequencies, is part of that spectrum.

When UVA strikes your skin, it penetrates deeply into the middle layer, the dermis. UVA alters your skin's DNA. It also causes photo-aging: the easily noticed premature blotchiness and wrinkling. UVB rays penetrate deep into the outer epidermis where it damages your cells and causes sunburn.

Almost all skin cancers are caused by over-exposure to sunlight. Ninety-five percent of all melanoma cases can be traced to over-exposure to sun. Ninety-nine percent of non-melanoma skin cancers are related to sun exposure.

There are three forms of skin cancer. The most common are basal cell carcinomas (BCCs). Nearly 3 million cases of BCCs are reported annually in the USA. Basal (meaning basic, or fundamental) cell carcinomas arise from the skin's outermost layer, the epidermis. Often disfiguring, but rarely life threatening, BCCs are found in areas with high levels of UV exposure. In general, for a cyclist, the hands, the nose, cheeks, eyelids, and the tips of the ears are most often the site of a BCC.

Squamous cell carcinomas (SCCs) are less common than BCCs. 700,000 cases of SCC are diagnosed each year in the US, but squamous (meaning covered in scales) cell carcinomas kill about 2,500 people each year. Located just above the basal cell layer of the skin, a cyclist might notice squamous damage by the classic signs of sun: wrinkling, changes in pigmentation, and loss of elasticity. Sun degrades the collagen which supports the skin. In my case, by the time melanoma struck, the backs of my hands looked like the bicycle tires I once raced upon.

Melanoma, the deadliest skin cancer, develops when your body can no longer repair the damage caused by UV radiation to its DNA. You should again recall from Bio 9 that in your DNA, the base thymine binds only to adenine and guanine binds only to cytosine. The initials A-T and C-G might look familiar. Repeated UV radiation encourages thymine to bind to another thymine and create thymine dimers. These dimers, the DNA base pair T-T, are bad things. Human DNA is very good at self-repair, but over time, the repair mechanism cannot keep up and your DNA is permanently damaged. As was mine.

I was now a mutant. The DNA mutations caused my skin cells to multiply rapidly and uncontrollably to form a malignant tumor. You must, by now, understand how DNA codes for everything, good and bad, in the body. I had melanoma. That's bad code.

Now, I had melanoma again, in the exact same place. My DNA was saying, "Sir, you are now programmed to have a tumor just in front of your left ear." I also understood that when cancer comes back, that's never good.

I was no longer concerned. I was scared.

The Second Freckle

Following Cath's discovery of the second lesion, my Tuesday 8:00 am phone call to Dr. Barkey's office the next morning had a different tone.

"Hi, this is David Stanley."

The receptionist heard a quavering sound. I squeaked like the voice of a 14-year-old boy calling to ask a girl to go to the dance with him.

"I'm one of Dr. Barkey's melanoma patients and I really need to meet with him as soon as possible because I have another lesion right on the same spot as the one that I had removed and I know that can't be a good thing so I need to get into the office right away. It's right in the same spot so this is kinda important so when can I have him look at it?"

I rambled. I rambled because that's what I do when I'm scared. I was now officially scared.

"Doctor gets here at 6:30 and keeps an early morning appointment for emergencies. Can you be here at 6:45 tomorrow morning? That's Wednesday," his receptionist asked.

I said, "Be there at 6:45? Hell, I'll camp out in the parking lot if I have to."

I pulled into the office parking lot right behind Dr. Barkey's assistant. I tapped on the steering wheel in time to the morning drive time radio's beat whilst I waited for the lights to come up and the front door to unlock. As the receptionist walked up to the door from the inside, I walked up from the outside.

As I signed in, I saw Dr. Barkey walk down a hall, a stack of charts in his hand. I could see he was reading. He bit his lower lip in concentration and walked into his office. He didn't see me.

The nurse led me back to an exam room, invited me in, and gestured towards a chair.

"He's on a phone call," she said. "He'll be with you right away."

I stood up from the exam chair to shake hands when Dr. Barkey walked into the room, still deep in the chart. He looked up. He had pursed lips. We shook hands. He nodded as he spoke.

"Dave," he said. "You know enough genetics to know that you must now have a serious genetic predisposition to melanoma in this spot. Let's have a look. Again, this is early. I really feel the need to repeat that."

I turned sideways. He put his magnifying lens over the spot.

"Hmm, *right on the old incision*. Hmm."

I could feel his breath on my ear.

"Well, we need to do another biopsy."

By now, I knew the drill. I would turn sideways. The nurse would adjust the headrest to properly support my head. The chair would tip down until parallel with the floor. I would have a pale blue drape placed over my face. She'd wipe my face with a sterilizing solution and set out Dr. Barkey's tools. One little needle stick, a touch of a burn, a scraping sound from the biopsy tool, and a band-aid. Chair rises.

Biopsy complete.

Dr. Barkey reminded me that this was still very early in the scheme of things. He reminded me that many people never have the *in situ* lesion. For most people with melanoma, this place where I now sat was exactly the spot from where most people with melanoma begin. He reminded me that it was far too early to allow any anxiety to affect my life. I played that tape in my head as I drove to school.

I taught my classes. I doubt my Wednesday classes were scintillating. Thursday's were certainly better. I had some time to think things through.

"Early detection is key," I said to myself.

"A smart guy's in charge," I reminded myself.

"It's still a very small lesion," I noted.

I was still apprehensive. The edge was gone from my anxiety.

The message light was blinking on my phone when I got home from teaching on Thursday.

"Dave, we need to meet tomorrow to discuss your treatment options. I held my morning 6:45 for you. Thanks. See you then."

This was delivered in a "Luke, I am your father, this is not open for discussion" voice.

When I awoke at 4:30 am, I realized that as Barkey's office was fifteen minutes away, I would have no trouble being there on time.

"Dave, you know your melanoma is back," Barkey said. "You also know that recurrence is not good. We're still early in this. You should have every confidence that you're going to be fine. That's why I'm sending you down to Ann Arbor. U-Hospital. Their Multi-Disciplinary Melanoma Clinic is the best in the world. And I'm not saying that just because I'm a die-hard Wolverine. Or that one of my best friends is the chief. But, being friends with Tim Johnson didn't hurt when I called down there about you. Call them when you get home and they'll see you next week."

"Next week?" I managed to stammer.

"Yes, next week. You are not in any dire straits, far from it. This is very slow growing stuff you have, Dave. You're going to be fine, but they need to get started. It might take a while to establish clean margins before the surgery."

"Margins?" I said. "They're not just taking the thing in front of my ear, then?"

"Let me explain a bit. It'll ease your mind a little, I think. This is pretty cool, actually. They'll do what's called a square procedure. You're familiar with Mohs surgery, right, where they take away bits of tissue at a time while you're in surgery until they get clear margins? This procedure has a better chance of establishing the margins prior to the big surgery. It's also better for necks and faces.

"They'll numb you up and then scribe, excise, with this neat double-bladed scalpel they invented, a very thin strip of skin, maybe two or three millimeters wide, all the way 'round your lesion. They'll suture you up and squirt some tattoo dye in there at the same time. Your students will think it's kind of cool. But they use the tattoo dye as markers. It'll be gone after the big surgery. You want a tattoo, you'll have to get your own."

"I think I'll pass on the tattoo," I said to Dr. Barkey. "There's something about a 50-year-old white guy getting a tattoo that seems a little too midlife crisis-ish to me. Thanks, though."

Dr. Barkey went on.

"Your tissue will go to the lab. If the margin for that side of the square is clean, no cancerous cells can be seen, they'll know how far out to go with the main surgery. If it's not clean, they scribe out further. It might take several go-rounds, you know. A couple weeks' worth of biopsies, okay, until they get four clean margins, one for each side of the square. Once they establish four clean and cancer-free margins, then they'll schedule the main surgery."

"Okay, then. They need to establish clean margins. I get that. But how much skin do you think…?" I asked.

"How much skin they will need to take, I can't tell," Barkey said. "Could be small; two, maybe three centimeters a side. But I'd plan on at least four centimeters the side. How deep? Well, that depends, too.

But pretty much, from the skin down, they'll scrape down to the bone. They want to take everything but the nerves and vessels. They can't leave anything behind."

"Leave anything behind?" I asked.

"Right. Here's why melanoma can be so dangerous. Melanoma likes to burrow. You know you've got all those lymph pathways in your neck. For a facial melanoma, that's like a freeway to your brain. They try to leave the skin, stretch it up over your surgical site like a facelift, but it depends on what the surgeon finds.

"You're not getting a real facelift, by the way. The surgeon will stretch the skin, if he can, but he won't do anything to anchor it place like a lift. So, you'll look kind of young on that side for a couple of months, but then you'll go back to your regular self. He may even need to do a graft from your hip or shoulder."

"A skin graft," I said. "That seems like they might be taking a big chunk of my face, then."

"A big chunk? Probably not, but I can't tell. Neither can they, until the margins are set. But they can't leave anything behind. So, good news, the odds are overwhelming that you'll be fine. The bad? Well, it could be a long summer. These guys are really good. They're the best. That's why I use them. They keep me posted on everything. You have any questions, call me. I'm easier to get to. I have a list up front of all my active patients. The women in front know to get me those calls ASAP.

"Look, it's early. All signs point in the right directions. I'm confident you're going to be okay."

I was confident. Scared, but confident.

Part Two
The Overture

Welcome to Ann Arbor

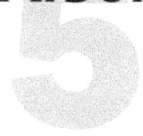

Ann Arbor is one of the Midwest's great cities. It is home to one of the world's finest research universities. The University of Michigan health care systems has so many groundbreaking programs that their Wikipedia page is 10,000 words and 40 pages long. A tour around town would take in Zingerman's food emporium, bits of an extraordinary music culture, and a visit to an arboretum and botanical garden known across the globe. Ann Arbor has a history of radical thought that many would argue gave birth to the anti-war movement of the 1960s, and enough weird denizens to keep a people-watcher happy for a long time.

It is also a city under constant construction, especially in the hospital zones. With an explosion of high-tech grant money and the donations of extremely wealthy alumni, a new wing or center or capital improvement seems always to be underway. In 2006, the time of my melanoma, GPS for the masses was in its infancy, and not entirely reliable. Couple this with the intermittent road closures for construction, and local knowledge was necessary.

Cath navigated. Cath lived in Ann Arbor for a dozen years. She graduated from the famed Rackham School of Graduate Studies. She worked for the University Hospital Systems. When it comes to Ann Arbor, she has a GPS in her frontal lobe. Parking, as in every urban campus environment, is on a wing and a prayer. As Cath says, "A parking permit at U of M is only a hunting license."

I drove. When I'm nervous, I have to drive. Of course, when I'm not nervous, I have to drive, too. Men. Driving. It's who we are.

I was not ready for the scene I saw when Cath and I got off the elevator for the Multidisciplinary Melanoma Clinic. These people were sick. Large pieces of face were missing. Entire mandibles, orbitals, ears, noses, sections of scalps. I worked in hospitals. I have taught human anatomy. I have dissected a cadaver. I was not ready for this. I rubbed my ear and plucked several stray hairs from my tragus. These people were now my peers. We all had melanoma.

Cath asked, "You alright?"

I was, I am certain, pasty-white. I looked around the waiting area again. My breath was shortened. My pulse accelerated. Up until this moment, my melanoma was an occasional speedbump on my road to wellness.

"I had a little thing," I thought. "I had it removed. A slightly bigger thing returned in its place. I'll get it removed, and boom, back to normal."

These people were the first tangible vision I had in which the melanoma was not defeated. These people, potentially, were my future. These people started out exactly like me.

"Yep, fine."

I lied. Cath knew I was lying. But at that moment of truth, as we both took in a potential future, telling her I was suddenly very scared didn't seem to have much utility. Anyone with cancer who came across the Multidisciplinary Melanoma Clinic waiting area, would be, *should be*, scared. I had the inarguable sensation that in an alternate universe, I was one of those brave people missing substantial amounts of facial bone and skin. So, I lied to my wife.

Truth is, I didn't have much choice but to act all right. The patient inventory ladies were waiting for me at one of the desks in a long row of cubbies.

One of the ladies called me over. She was a serenely placid woman. She gestured softly, to indicate we should take a seat.

"Um, no thanks," I said. "Probably better if I stand."

She smiled. Tranquil. Her mood was like Xanax.

"I understand. We get that a lot."

She looked at Cath and smiled.

"It's always the men."

Seated in front of her screen, she ran through my history with me, forwarded by Dr. Barkey's office. They knew I severed a wrist tendon from a ski injury in 1976. They knew I'd had knee surgery in college from a soccer injury in 1978. They knew I'd burst a bursa in my elbow from a bike racing accident in 1986. And a broken collarbone from another bike racing accident in 1988. They knew I'd had a chronic fatigue disease that lasted three months: cytomegalovirus, in 1994. I nodded in agreement as she ran through my list of injuries and illnesses, nearly all of them the result of pilot error.

I swear that jasmine and honeysuckle were wafting out of her computer. I could feel my blood pressure return to its normal, non-adrenalized state. I was aware that I could no longer feel my heartbeat thumping in my ears.

She reached for my hand.

I must have looked terribly startled.

She stopped and showed me what she had in her other hand.

"ID bracelet?"

Her eyes smiled. I do believe that on the inside, she was about to figuratively shoot Ovaltine out her nose but was far too gentle a soul to do so. She handed me a card. A maize and blue U-M hospital ID card.

"You'll need that every time you return for treatment or a consult. Oh, and did you park in the ramp? We validate, you know. Why don't you head over towards the intake desk? The nurse will come for you over there."

I chuckled.

She cocked her head to the side and raised an eyebrow, questioning.

"You validate. It just struck me funny. Here we are, this cancer center, all these sick people, and still, everyone is pretty stoked to get free parking in Ann Arbor. Kinda funny."

She looked at me and smiled.

"I hear the couch is pretty comfy."

We sat, Cath and I. The couch was comfy. Not too cushy. I was seated just long enough to pull out a copy of *Outside* from inside my backpack. I leaned back and crossed my legs with the casual, devil-may-care insouciance which belongs to all cancer patients. At that very moment, a woman in scrubs, holding a chart, and bearing a perky smile came at a near-trot from the hallway into the vestibule near "our" couch.

"Mr. Stanley? David Stanley?"

And boom, blood pressure, thumping in my ears, right back up where it belonged.

I found myself singing:

> *Bad boys, bad boys whatcha gonna do?*
> *Whatcha gonna do when they come for you?*
> *Bad boys, bad boys whatcha gonna do?*
> *Whatcha gonna do when they come for you?*

They were here and they were here for me. Cath and I followed her down the hall. If they had rolled me, at that very instant, into an MRI machine, the singularly recognizable mixture of hospital smell and pervasive fear was so deep into my brain that both of my olfactory lobes and my amygdalae would have lit up like fireworks on the Fourth of July. We walked into a large exam room, dimly lit and very quiet.

We sat, the three of us. The nurse checked my card. She checked my wrist band. She checked my vitals. My pulse, normally a tortoise-like 52 to 56, was racing in the 90s like a hamster on wheel. My blood pressure, normally a soporific 110/70, was now galloping along at 150/90.

"You don't have a history of high blood pressure, do you?" she asked.

"No, never. My vitals usually weird people out 'cause they head in the opposite direction," I said.

"Nervous?" she asked.

"Nah, not really," I said.

She raised an eyebrow at me.

"Um, yeah, I'm totally lying to you. I'm mostly scared shitless and trying not to get up and run around the room," I said.

"We get that a lot," she said. "And please, don't go for your run now. It scares the other patients. I beg you."

She looked at Cath.

"It's always the men," said the nurse. "Just kidding. It's everybody. This is a scary time. It's okay."

"Vitals aside, what you're seeing is pretty normal." Cath said. "He's usually a pretty calm guy, but when my husband gets wound up, he gets really wound up. You've been warned."

"Don't go anywhere," the nurse said. "The rest of team will be here in a moment. I'll be right back," she said.

"I'll be right here. I'm not going anywhere."

She smile, turned, and left the room.

"Where the Hell else would I go?" I thought. "I'm sitting here with melanoma. Again."

A Handsome Young Doctor

I told the nurse I wouldn't go anywhere. I told her I wouldn't go for a run. I did not tell her I would sit down. Under the best of times, I am rarely successful at stillness. This may not have been the worst of times, but it was clearly not the best of times.

Cath sat in silence as I wandered the exam room. I became expert with the warning signs of skin cancer, as advertised by surgical instrument company posters on the walls. I memorized the labels on the drawers. I investigated the suction canisters hanging on the walls. I admired the heft and feel of the curtain which could be pulled around the exam chair. I was reading the warning label on the sharps container, my back to the room, when I heard the shuffle of many feet in the doorway. I did a quick hop, a 180 degree turn. There was a cadre of folks standing in the doorway.

"Oh, hey! Hi!" I said.

Hail fellow well met, I faked good cheer and happiness. The group was led by a tall, sturdy man, mid-thirties, quite handsome in an "I rowed crew as an undergrad" sort of way. Four or five followers stood behind him.

"G'day, mate! How are you today, Mr. Stanley?" he said, in a perfect Down Under accent. "I'm Dr. Ludgate. Matt Ludgate."

"What part of Oz are you from?" I asked.

"Oz? No, mate. I'm Kiwi, through and through. Auckland. Don't ever make that mistake again."

He laughed. There was laughter, in a world-renowned cancer clinic, in my exam room. I took this as a good sign.

"You're one of Dr. Barkey's patients. He's one of our best referrings."

Doing my best Clint Eastwood, I squinted up at him. From my 5'6" it was quite a distance.

"Best referrings? There's that much work? Well, crap."

He laughed again.

"C'mon, mate. Lighten up. I mean, when Barkey sends us a patient, we get always get a great report. Good history, spot-on labs. He's a good man, Barkey. That's what I mean.

"Lots of sun exposure, Barkey says, when you were younger? Raced bicycles, spent lots of time in Texas? I rode a lot, mountain bikes, to keep fit for rugby. Played a lot of rugger at school. Fly-half, that was me."

The fly-half position, near the scrum, the central moving hillock of players, is a bit like the quarterback in American football. The fly-half is typically the orchestrator of the offense and the director of defense. He's called upon to sprint, tackle, pass, and think in the midst of rugby madness. I also chose to take this as a good sign.

"I played a bit of rugby in college; scrum-half," I said. "Do you still play?"

He looked like he could still play.

"Not really, mate. Weekend laughers is all. I'm busy. Can't you tell I'm in demand?" he said as he waved his hand at his acolytes.

He laughed at himself.

This Ludgate bloke was good. I was calmer. He had "established rapport."

"I know Dr. Barkey has explained what we're going to do, but I'd like to go over it again, just so I understand that you understand. Be patient with me."

"I'll do my best."

It was my turn to laugh.

"Here ya go, mate. Have a seat," he said and pointed to the end of the exam table.

I hopped onto the end of the table whilst Ludgate settled himself in a rolling chair. I glanced at Cath in the room's padded armchair. She was quiet.

Dr. Ludgate caught my glance. He turned.

"I'm sorry. Mrs. Stanley? I'm Dr. Ludgate. I should have introduced myself straightaway. My apologies."

He smiled. His teeth gleamed. Cath smiled back. He was handsome.

"Not a problem, Doctor. Don't let me stop you," she replied.

Ludgate turned back towards me.

"Right, so off we go. You have a 1.5-centimeter recurrent lesion just in front of your left ear's tragus, that little nub in front of your ear canal. See, I did read your chart this morning."

We both laughed.

"It was biopsied, came back positive, and removed as *in situ*, which is good, last year. But it returned, in the same spot, and not, *not*, hmm, *in situ*, one year later. This, you know, is *not* a good thing. Today, we are going to start the work for a square procedure. What we do is, we scribe, well, we scribe a rough square around the lesion. Each side of the square is a tissue sample 1–2 millimeters wide and about 4 centimeters long. We color-code each side by squirting a bit of tattoo dye into the biopsy area and then stitch you up. We use blue and red. I'll alternate colors so we can tell which end goes where.

"If you'd like something else, something that might match your wardrobe or hair color, I'll see what we have. The tattoos are temporary anyway. The surgeon who does the final procedure uses my tattoo lines as his guideline for the removal of the lesion.

"We'll send the tissue samples to the lab and they'll read them off, see if we have clean margins, no signs of cancerous or pre-cancerous cells. Dr. Barkey explained how melanoma sends out little runners, little threads, mate, of pre-cancerous tissue?"

I nodded.

"He explained how, untreated, melanoma can create brain metastases, yes? I'll bet he said 'melanoma likes to go home to the brain?'"

I laughed and nodded. "Exactly. That's exactly what he said."

"Well, it's a pretty accurate phrase. That's why melanoma in your location is potentially, remember, I'm saying potentially, without treatment, so dangerous?"

I nodded again.

"Excellent," the doctor said.

"Right-o, mate. So, we hear back from the lab. If a side is clean, we leave it alone. If we don't have a clean margin, we scribe that side again, longer this time, and further away from your original lesion…"

I interrupted. "But, how do you know how far away, how long…"

"Exactly, Mr. Stanley. Good point. That's what I get paid for. Partly, it's my experience. I do these a lot. I'm in my second year post-doc here. I do six or eight of these every day, three or four days a week. That's why I'm here; to do as many as I can. I compare final margins with initial margins, so I develop, a, er, a sort of feel. That and sometimes just blind luck, mate.

"So, anyway, we keep bringing you back until we establish four clean margins. We could hit it straightaway, but I'll be honest, that's rare. It's usually two or three tries 'til everything is clean. Once we're clean all around, we send you to the derm surgeon who specializes in these. You'll have a consult and then he goes to work.

"All told, today's biopsy will run about an hour. We have to do another? They run a bit shorter, yes? We'll have less cutting to do. The final surgery? That's up to the surgeon, but figure 3–6 hours, depending.

He's not just good at clearing out the cancer, this guy, but he's a top shelf plastics guy, too. You'll look pretty when he's done."

The doc tilted his head and looked at me a little cock-eyed. It was his turn to squint hard now. He looked over at Cath: my wife, an RN, BSN, MSN. She was sitting over to one side, completely silent, taking it all in.

He smiled from ear to ear at her. It was a very winning smile.

"Well, Mrs. Stanley, he won't look any worse. Promise."

He turned back to me.

I suspect I still looked like I'd seen a ghost.

"Geez, mate, I mean, Mr. Stanley. Lighten up. You got this. It's early. We're good. You're gonna be fine.

"Let's get this started."

Panic in Ann Arbor

"I'm glad he's confident," I thought. "Easy for Ludgate. It's not his face."

His crew looked up at him. Feet shuffled. Papers rustled and shifted in this pre-iPad chart era.

"Okay, Mr. Stanley..." he said.

I interrupted.

"Dave. Let's go with Dave, okay? We're going to be kind of intimate, right? What with you breathing in my ear and invading my face with a scalpel and all? We should probably be on a first name basis."

"Right. Good idea. Let's begin again. I'm Matthew Ludgate. Matt."

He towered over me as he drew himself to his full height. He stood at attention, arms tucked at his sides, chin in, chest out and announced in a stentorian voice, "Dr. Ludgate, sir. I'll be doing your biopsy today."

We both burst out laughing. I heard Cath's laughter.

In his normal voice he said, "It's time to get started. I need to check on a patient in the next room. Be back in ten minutes and we'll get going."

He waved and walked out.

The nurse gestured to me.

"Okay, Mr. Stanley. Time to do this. I'll prep you, numb you up, and then buzz Dr. Ludgate. Okay?"

My blood pressure went from normal to redlined in 1.6 seconds.

"Whoa, Whoa, Whoa! Numb me up!! You're a nurse. Don't take this the wrong way, but I've worked in hospitals, I mean, anesthesia? That's a doctor thing. I'm sure you're really good at derm nursing, but I've been stitched up and had a lot of surgery, and doctors always..."

She smiled at me. It was a sympathetic smile. I seemed to get a lot of those smiles on this day.

Cancer; it gets your adrenalin running. At this moment, mine had me 3 seconds away from a 50-meter dash out the door and down the hall to the stairwell.

"That's true, Mr. Stanley.

"Are we on a first name basis, too? Dave, you're right, every other hospital I've worked at, docs always did their own anesthesia. But here, because of the way the patients flow through the clinic, nurses do the biopsy anesthesia. It was Dr. Johnson's idea, you know, the clinic director. He had to sell the Board on it.

"He convinced them by having a few of us numb him up at a Board meeting. Good move, huh? Look, he was just around the corner. I'll grab if him for you, if I can."

She held up one finger.

"Don't go anywhere, okay? Promise? Be right back."

She smiled, and darted out the door.

She walked back in with the clinic director, Dr. Tim Johnson.

He walked over to me and stuck out his hand.

"I'm Tim Johnson. They kind of let me run this place. I hear you're one of Walt Barkey's guys. Walt and I go way back. Tell me, he still have that Audi TT? Nice car."

I nodded. I tried to smile.

I blurted out, "Yes, he does. You're right. Nice car. Hey, I'm wondering…"

"Right. You're wondering about your anesthesia."

He nodded at the nurse.

"They're good. They're better than any resident that ever worked on you in an ER, I promise you. They had to be, for me to sell the Medical Practices Board. They're all great nurses, and they know how to give injections. I trained them, along with a couple of our anesthesia guys who work with our clinic. After we were certain of their skills, I took them into a meeting. They numbed my arm. We did a little biopsy, just like the one you had. Then another nurse numbed a different spot. One of the post-docs did a little incision, like the one you're having, and then stitched me up. Look, I still have the scar."

He pushed up the sleeve of his lab coat. He had a scar, three-quarters of an inch long and a millimeter or two wide, on his forearm. I looked at his arm, then up at him. He smiled with pride.

"The Board was pretty shocked, I tell you, when we did that. But our nurses are good. They're really good. They don't work here, otherwise."

He smiled again.

The nurse glowed.

I smiled.

"Where'd you get this idea?" I asked. "Don't people think it's weird? I mean, I'm fine with it. Now, I mean, after you've explained it, but I've spent a lot of time in hospitals. I've never seen this before."

"Not so much. Health care providers notice. People like you—people who spend a lot of time in ER—you guys notice. But this way, our clinic is way more efficient. The docs practice better medicine. They see more people. We use more of our nurses' skills, too.

"Look, we're going to take good care of you. All of us. I promise. Tell Walt I said hi, wouldja? Tell him I checked in on you."

I breathed deeply and lay back, on my side, in the exam chair. It was not uncomfortable. The nurse leaned in and looked at the side of my face. Her breath was cooler than Ludgate's. I could smell her hair.

She stood back, flipped through my chart and asked me to re-state my allergies.

I sat up.

"Biaxin, Ceclor, and bee stings," I said.

She nodded.

"But no allergy issues with local anesthesia?"

"Well, I'm pretty sensitive to epi."

Epi, short for epinephrine, is adrenalin—the "fight or flight" hormone. Epinephrine is often added to local anesthesia as a vasoconstrictor to slow down the rate at which the local anesthesia is absorbed. In short, it makes the anesthesia last longer.

"What happens to you?" she asked.

"Well, if I just need a couple of stitches, or whatever, it's no big deal, but like if need to have a wisdom tooth pulled, when they shoot the Novocain in, I could pretty much run a 40-second 400 meters, you know? I found out the hard way a few years back. My oral surgeon liked to use a lot, and it hit me all at once, and man, I tell you, it took all I've got not to rip the arms off his dentist chair, and maybe the dentist, too. So, um, yeah…kind of a problem."

Even thinking back to my last wisdom tooth removal was enough to get my panic level back to Defcon 2.

"Let me note that," she said. "We need to use a lot, too, so, well, um, we can use the epi-free solution. The epi, you know, helps hold the Novocain in place, and you're going to have a pretty big field, so we'll probably have to give you a few extra shots along the way. If that's okay with you, then that's what I'll do."

"Better a few little needle sticks, I think, than you needing to put me in restraints, so, yeah, epi-free sounds great."

I leaned back, breathing deeply again.

The nurse reached behind her, towards the counter, and took down a Sharpie and a small flexible, plastic ruler.

"It's how we mark the edge of the margins. Dr. Ludgate wants to start with a 5-centimeter square around your lesion."

I felt first the ruler and then, the Sharpie, as she traced a square, two inches per side, around that odd freckle directly in front of my left tragus.

She turned to the counter behind her, reached for a bottle of anesthetic and began to draw the first of several syringes of the clear liquid. I watched her. She inserted the last needle into the bottle. She watched me watching her.

"Nervous?" she asked. "About the anesthesia, I mean. I know you're nervous about the biopsy and melanoma and all."

"Nah, I'm good. I've had lots of stitches," I said. "Novocain's no big deal. Gotta like the epi-free version, though. I'll be asking for that at the dentist, that's for sure."

She laughed as she leaned in.

"You'll feel a needle stick, a little sting, right? You know how this goes. After the first stick, I work out from the numb spot so you won't feel the needle sticks from then on. This will take a few minutes."

Slowly, from a spot down near my left earlobe, past my tragus and up in front of my ear, across the base of my sideburn, down the margin of my zygomatic arch—the bone that articulates with the back end of the mandible—and then back up to my ear lobe, I felt a cooling numbness in the shape of a trapezoid fill in across the side of my face. I reached up and touched my cheek. Wooden.

I heard a scuffling sound in the doorway. I didn't think I should move so I rolled my eyes up a bit in my head so I could catch a glimpse of the door. Ludgate and his entourage were back.

"Dave-o," he announced, "I think we are ready."

He put on a mask. He was already wearing a surgical cap. I noticed his crew was standing well behind him. He took a pair of gloves from the counter and pulled them on. As he interlaced his fingers to set the gloves fully on his hands, the gloves squeaked like kids playing with balloons.

He sat himself down at my side, near my head. I could see him, if I strained my vision, reach for the parallel-bladed biopsy scalpel.

He turned to his nurse.

"Perfect. This looks perfect. Nice work."

He turned back to my cheek.

"Okay? Okay," he murmured.

As the scalpel pushed through my skin, I heard the sound of a kitchen cleaver being dragged across the plate glass window of my skull.

The Kindness of Strangers

I was ready for discomfort. I have been poked, prodded, splinted, and stitched in emergency rooms and operating room suites across North America. Admittedly, when I get a cold, I am a giant sissy. However, as a ski racing goalkeeping bicycle racer, I proudly take my lumps and come back for more. Every scar is a story. Every lump left behind from a broken bone is a badge of honor. I am out there; taking risks and living life. As Patrick Swayze's character Dalton says in *Road House*, "Pain don't hurt."

The shriek of that scalpel cutting through my face, however, was a sound effect for which I was entirely unprepared. It was, in the most visceral fashion imaginable, utterly terrifying. It was the slam of a prison cell door for a crime I didn't commit. It was fingers on a blackboard. It was grinding teeth. It was the squeak of a knife against a china plate at 110 decibels in a dark, cobwebbed room. It was an explosion on a jet liner as oxygen masks fell from the ceiling. It was dread.

Until that moment, I tried to be rational with my cancer. I viewed it as an outsider. The research said this intruder was easy to handle. In my analytical brain, I described the procedure to the rest of my mind, and put matters, I believed, to rest. With the sound of the knife cutting 1–2 millimeters, the thickness of a dime, down into the skin of my face, directly in front of my ear, my reptilian brain let out one gigantic "What the fuck is going on here?"

I believe I paled. I know I paled. I may have gasped. Or shouted. I gurgled as I desperately tried to avoid vomiting into the back of my mouth.

Dr. Ludgate stopped cutting for a moment.

"Dave-o? Everything okay?"

"Okay? Um, yeah. No. Er, I don't know what…"

"Take a few deep breaths, wouldja please? You're scaring my nurse. Kinda bothering me a wee bit, too, if I tell the truth."

David L. Stanley

His students lined the wall behind him. I could see their reflections. They stood stock-still, like the terracotta warriors and horses sculptures that depict the armies that even in death protect Qin Shi Huang, the first emperor of China. I took a few deep breaths. My lesion was directly in front of my ear. I understood what was happening: bone conduction. While it is true that much of our hearing results from sound waves causing deflections in the eardrum, a sizeable amount of hearing also results from bone conduction. The sound waves strike the skin and bone of your skull. Much like a drumhead, the slightest tap echoes within your ear canal.

Have you ever placed your ear against a wooden 2 x 4 and had someone very gently scratch the other end of the 2 x 4? You hear it quite clearly, don't you? In fact, sound travels nearly ten times faster through wood than it does through air. The skin and bone around your ears are also quite good conductors of sound. Bone conduction—the barely audible sound of scalpel gently cutting through skin was being amplified, like a drum head, through the skin near my ear, and rocketing into my ear canal. It was as if South Africa had won soccer's World Cup and all that country's vuvuzela horns went off in my head at once. I sorted all this out in a few moments. Rationality didn't help.

"Hey, um, Matt? Kind of need a moment here, okay?"

"That hurt?" Dr. Ludgate asked.

He sounded surprised.

"Oooh, no. It's great. I've had lots of stitches, surgeries. We're good there. She did great. You're doing great. No, I just need to, ah, catch my breath for a second. Right?"

"Well, what's up then? Maybe I can, you know, help things along?"

"Well, Matt, I'm not sure how, I mean, how to say this, but um, it sounds in here, you know, inside my head, like the top of my head is getting cut off with a chainsaw. I'll, uh, cut to the chase here."

Deep breath.

"Matt, it's scaring the piss out of me."

"Ah. Yes. Well, that makes sense, mate. I mean, I am working right in front of your ear. Right? How about if I just chat with you a bit while I work, and you, well, I can't really have you answer much, your jaw wiggles when you talk and I am working near your T-M joint, so I'll talk and if you need a moment, just hold up a finger and we'll take a quick break. Sound good? Any pain? No? Good. Let me know if you want more local. Without the epi, the local wears off quicker. Okay? Good. Here we go.

"So, you said you played soccer?" Back to work for Dr. Ludgate.

Back to Zen breathing for me. One. Two. Three. Four. And again.

58

As he finished the careful extraction of each strip of skin, Ludgate placed it in a glass tray filled with preservative. In my histochemistry classes at Michigan State, I had worked for a professor doing research on testicular cancer. I had done much the same procedure to lab rats. Dead lab rats.

He stitched as he went, carefully joining the sides of his 2-millimeter wide, 2-millimeter deep, 5-centimeter long incisions. As he stitched, I could hear the squish squash of the tattoo dye bottle as he marked his work with either red or blue dye.

"That's it, mate. We're done. Good on ya'! Made it. Want to see?"

"Yeah. Sure. Lemme see."

Now that we were finished, my rational brain was back in charge.

Dr. Ludgate's assistant held up a tray which held several small glass containers. In each were the ultra-thin strips of skin he had just removed; all labeled for location and all color-coded in red or blue.

"Nice," I said. "That is very cool."

"Can I see my face?"

"Sure. We need pictures anyway. Sit up a bit straighter. Don't move. Smile. Just kidding. Don't smile. Smiles'll move your skin. Hold it."

Hummm. Click. "Done."

He held out the camera. I had a 2-inch square scribed on the side of my face, outlined in alternating red and blue dye, directly in front of my tragus. His stitchwork was small, neat and precise. The square looked pretty cool, aside from the fact that it was on my face, and it outlined my cancer. On the other hand, it also outlined the sector of my cheek the surgeon would remove as he prevented the cancer from eroding away my face.

Dr. Ludgate said, "Here's what we do. These samples go the lab where they are read by a skin cancer specialist. That's all they do, read samples from skin cancer biopsies. Our pathologists are very good. Very good, indeed.

"If a margin, an incision, is clean, no cancerous and pre-cancerous cells seen, then we're done with that side. If not, we get instructions from the lab on how far back we should push the next margin, if we should lengthen the margin. And we repeat the process. This way, we have the best chance to get all of the cancer and pre-cancerous cells in one swoop."

"How do they know," I asked, "how far back to move the margin?"

"Right," Ludgate said. "About that. If they see a large number of pre-cancerous cells, they tell me to move it back a fair amount. If just few are seen, histologically, then they tell me to move it back just a bit. Experience, mostly, Dave. They do these a lot. We're pretty busy. They see a lot of cases and they can track their recommendations against their outcomes. Data, mate."

I reached up and tapped the side of my face. I could feel the little brush-like projections of his needlework. The stitches felt familiar. Without thinking, I tapped my tragus in front of my ear. Ludgate saw me.

"Yes. Your ear. I don't know, at least until we get the labs back, how far back the pre-cancerous cells might go. My gut tells me that your ear is probably safe. Probably. That's not a promise. I mean, you have melanoma near your ear."

I interrupted.

"My ear. Right, I get that. But what about my hearing? What's the likelihood that, even if everything goes pretty well, that I might lose some hearing? Or even all my hearing? I mean, I like my ear, but it's not the outside I'm all that worried about. What about the inside stuff?"

"That, Dave-O is something I can't tell you. With where we are now, as far as your lesion and its possible damage is concerned, I really don't know what might happen with your hearing itself. I am slightly concerned about the aesthetics of your outer ear.

"But your hearing itself? You know that most of your hearing is deep inside the skull, right? So, if, and this is an enormous if, you do suffer some hearing loss as a result, you're going to have plenty of other issues on your plate. Again, no guarantees mate, you know that, but based on my experience, and the literature on melanoma in this location, I have no reason to believe your hearing is at risk."

I nodded. I knew what "plenty of other issues" meant. It meant my lesion had metastasized and become lesions, plural, in my brain. Brain mets, in the medical vernacular.

"So don't worry about that. Try to not worry about your external ear, either. It's too soon to worry about it. When I tell you to worry? That's the time to worry. Right?

"Normally, we get the labs back in a few days. Your skin has several days of prep work ahead of it before the pathologists can read it. We'll be in touch by the end of the week, latest."

We packed up and went home. I drove. Now laden with nervous energy, it would have been wiser to bring my bike and do a fifty mile training ride from Ann Arbor back to Flint.

I had been cautioned about not training hard.

"Don't let your heart rate get up there too high," Dr. Ludgate had said. "We don't want a lot of blood pumping through there with all the cutting we've done. Ride. Lift. Run. Whatever you do, keep doing it. It'll keep you sane. But, and I can't stress this enough: Mate, you gotta take things easy. Get it?"

"Yes, sir."

I heard Cath from across the room.

"He'll take things easy, Dr. Ludgate. I promise."

"Thank you, Mrs. Stanley. I worked hard on this. We can't have your husband messing up my work."

In the car on the way home, Cath, a pensive look on her face, also urged me to relax.

"You need to take this as it comes. You can't just go into your frantic hyperspace mode here. This is going to be a long process. I know you. I know you're going to try and out-work this, stay ahead of it, somehow adrenalize this thing out of your system. You know that won't work. So try to be a little mellow with this, okay?"

She was 100% right, of course. I, however, had no ability to heed her advice.

Immediately upon returning home, I decided I needed to do the grocery shopping.

Cath sighed.

I was standing in the cereal aisle, choosing which Chex cereal we needed, when an older woman pushing her cart with a boy, perhaps six or seven, in the kid seat, came down the aisle. They stopped near me.

The kid was looking at me. He was holding a small stuffed dinosaur.

I looked back at him.

Stand-off.

I waved.

He looked down at his dino. He looked back at me.

"What's wrong with your face?" he asked.

Not loud. Not rude. Truly curious, with the innocent manner that only small kids can be curious.

I reached up and touched the side of my face.

Grandmother shushed him.

Loudly.

"You mean this?" I asked.

I touched my square.

"Uh-huh," he said.

He was staring, jaws agape.

I looked at his grandmother.

"Can I talk to him?"

She nodded.

"I have cancer on my face. That means some of my skin isn't working right. So, the doctors will remove the bad skin and good skin will grow in its place."

"It's blue," he said.

"True enough. That's so the doctors know where to take away the bad skin. It's red, too."

"Hey, yeah! That's cool!" he said.

True enough, I thought.

In the check-out line, I noticed a woman stealing glances at my ear. She leaned forward and, in a half-whisper, said, "I'm sorry. Excuse me. Can I ask: square procedure?"

"Um, yeah, how did you…?"

She slid the top of her T-shirt away from her neck. There was a nicely healed wound, about four inches by two inches, running under her bra strap and out to the edge of her shoulder.

"I was a lifeguard."

She shrugged.

"You must be at U-M, right? You're going to be fine. They're really nice down there. I'll pray for you."

"Thank you," I said. "That's very nice of you. I appreciate it."

As we stood in the check-out line at Kroger, she reached across and patted my arm. Her hand was warm on this June day. I wanted to hug her. I didn't. I should have.

Standing in line with this kind woman, I didn't feel the need to state that I didn't believe in the power of intercessory prayer. What I got was a warm feeling, that it wasn't just me and Cath and the family in this. It was everybody. All of us are touched by cancer. Some 600,000 US citizens die of cancer every year. Another fourteen million of us, every year, live with cancer. In Kroger, inside of fifteen minutes, I was reminded that from kid to grown-up, it's a fight we fight together. Like Red Green says on his PBS television show, "Remember, I'm pullin' for you. We're all in this together."

At dinner that night, Aaron asked, "So, how'd it go?"

"Not bad," I said. "I'll find out in a few days if I need another biopsy."

"Not bad?" said Cath. "You did great."

With a glance at Cath, I related to Aaron the story of my two meltdowns and the biopsy procedure.

"So, Dad, pretty much normal, then?" he asked.

"Yessir, pretty much normal."

Several days later, the phone rang.

"Mr. Stanley. This is the U-M Melanoma Clinic. We have your lab results back. Two of your margins are clear. The other two are not.

"We have several openings next week for your next biopsy. Do you have your calendar handy?

Scary Monster

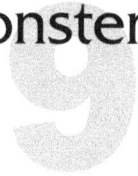

The appointment was made for a Tuesday. If one has to get melanoma, it's good to be a public school teacher. There is a 25% chance of scheduling one's health care crisis around summer vacation. I may not get paid for three months of the summer, but I didn't have to use any sick days either.

Ann Arbor is an especially lovely town in summer. Most of the undergrad students are gone. That means parking and traffic and restaurant seating are at tolerable levels. Ann Arbor is so lovely that we invited my father Mort, a retired physician, along for the ride. He spent his medical career doing family practice and proctology.

I thought he might be interested in watching the procedure. If I was not the patient, I believe I'd have been very interested. My university histochemistry background nurtured a strong interest in all things tissue and pathological. But on the basis of watching a biopsy, Mort was only marginally interested in making the trip.

Cath came a bit stronger. She bribed him with a post-biopsy pastrami sandwich at Zingerman's: quite possibly the world's finest delicatessen and food shrine not located in New York or Paris.

The drive was quiet. Cath read. Mort dozed. NPR droned low and ignored in the background; something about a meteor impact in Norway and sanctions against Iran and a Supreme Court ruling on medical marijuana. With no effective chemotherapy for melanoma, and hence no nausea, marijuana was of no interest to me. I'm in favor of sanctions against all theocracies. A meteor anywhere, even 3,800 miles away would normally be of interest, but today, my interest was centered on the 20 square centimeters of my face directly in front of my left ear. Absent-mindedly, I flicked the stubs of my sutures back and forth as I drove.

Cath, Dave and Mort arrived at the clinic with an ace up our sleeve—Mort's handicapped parking hang tag. My father had a quadruple cardiac bypass and still deals with a reasonable amount of claudication in his calf. Walking any distance over uneven terrain is often a chore. After 70 minutes of inactivity as a passenger, walking over pavement could be a too-painful chore. His tag allowed us to park a lob wedge away from the door. A 30-yard walk, a short hop up the elevator to the second floor, and directly to the back desks. It occurred to me that I now knew the way.

"We're regulars," I thought. "We get to skip the hoi polloi milling around out front and head directly to the VIP room."

Another charming and perky nurse led my father and me back to an exam room.

I introduced my father to the nurse. I explained that he was my dad, and a retired physician. Cath, wisely, chose to sit this one out. Two Stanley men were quite enough for the staff to handle.

"Where do they get these women?" I thought, as she chatted with my Dad about his practice. "Do they guide the best and the brightest of the cheerleading squad directly into dermatology nursing?"

She offered my Dad the comfy chair in the corner of the room whilst I hopped onto the exam table. I offered my arm for the blood pressure cuff. She wrapped the cuff around my upper arm, pumped up the sphygmomanometer and placed her stethoscope against my arm. I could feel my pulse pounding down my forearm and out into my fingertips. I also felt a weak twitch in my left eyelid. I heard the slow whoosh of the air flowing out the valve.

She frowned, tilted her head, and said, "There's nothing in your chart about high blood pressure. Are you feeling a bit nervous?"

Thinking I was answering truthfully, I shook my head and said, "Uh, no. I feel fine. Really."

She looked at me over the top of her glasses. "Really?"

"Yeah, I'm good. No worries. I got this."

Glancing at the cuff still on my arm, she said, "I've got a reading that says otherwise."

From behind us, a gruff voice from the comfy chair, "Whaddaya got?"

"156 over 96, Doctor."

A laugh, somewhere between a chortle and guffaw, came from Mort. "You're full of crap, David Stanley."

"Um, okay. Sure, I'm a little nervous. I mean, well, um. Ah, shit. Yeah, I hate this."

The nurse looked at me, kindly, and said, "That, Mr. Stanley, is what we usually hear around here. Thank you."

She made some notes on the chart. As she left the room, she said, "Doctor will be here in a few moments, and then his nurse will get started on your anesthetic."

I raised a hand to halt her. "I have an…"

She interrupted. "Epinephrine sensitivity. Right. We know. It's in your chart." She stuck the chart in the cubby outside the exam room door, waved, and was gone.

My father is a pacer. One of my earliest childhood family vacation memories is the time we were stuck in traffic for some time. As the accident cleared, we pulled into the rest stop so we could all "rest." My dad, a high school track star, ran several sprints around the parking lot to "loosen up."

I have inherited my Dad's pacing. Seated there on the exam table, I wanted to get up and, once again, check out the posters and drawer signage. Mort, however, had beaten me to it. As I sat, and watched my Dad read signs from drug companies about the warning signs of a variety of skin cancers, a new doctor wandered into the room.

He was my height; short. He was very slight. He walked into the exam room, nodded silently at me, opened a chart at the computer station, and logged in.

"Whatcha doing?" I asked.

"Reading this chart," he answered. He bent forward over the terminal.

A quiet man, no doubt.

I hopped off the exam table and skittered over to him like a gecko closing on a housefly. I stopped closer to him than perhaps normal social distances would allow.

"You're not Dr. Ludgate. I thought Dr. Ludgate would be doing my biopsy. Who are you?" I demanded.

I suspect my body language resembled Marvelous Marvin Hagler in his middleweight heyday at a weigh-in.

"I don't think I'm okay with this," I stammered.

"Where's Ludgate? He's the guy who does my biopsies!"

I could feel my pulse pounding in my ears.

The doctor took several nervous steps backwards.

"I'm not sure where Dr. Ludgate is at the moment. I can ask a nurse to find him for you. I just stopped in to use the work station. I'm sorry to have disturbed you. I, uh, I'll go now."

He took another backwards step away from me, turned, and headed quite briskly down the hall to the left.

I was still standing there, staring down the hall, when I heard a shuffling of feet behind me from the other end of the hall.

It was Dr. Ludgate and his entourage.

"Down Bessy!! What was all that rot about?"

I must have looked startled.

"You were shouting at him, Dave-o."

Ludgate looked down at me. He did not look pleased.

I looked at my Dad. Mort snickered, nodded.

I shrugged.

"Oops. I should probably go apologize…" I started down the hall.

"No worries, mate. I'll talk to him later. If you went after him now, he might call security on you, thinking you're for real. It's only a scratch, right? I'll take care of it. You're not the first mate to go nanas around here.

"Nervous?"

I lay there on the table, face numb, with a new pair of Sharpie lines on my face. Two lines would stay untouched. Those two tattooed and stitched lines were free of pre-cancerous cells. They marked the edge of the clean margins. One line was just a few millimeters in front of my tragus and it paralleled my sideburn. It went from my hairline down towards the temporomandibular joint of my jaw.

The other tattooed line intersected the top of the tragal line. It started several centimeters above my tragus and continued at a slight angle for 7–8 centimeters. If you would have drawn a continuous straight line from where it stopped, it would have met the corner of my eye.

The new Sharpie lines were longer than before. When Sharpies draw slowly across your face, the cooling effect as the solvent evaporates and the dye leaves its mark behind is quite remarkable. The new lines marked out uncharted territory. They also were appreciably further away from the lesion than the original lines. Those two Sharpie lines would determine how much of my face would ultimately be excised. I lay still.

I may not believe in intercessory prayer but I did wish magical thoughts that Ludgate would hit these two new margins spot-on. I could still hear the shrieking of that damned scalpel bouncing around inside my skull. This time, it sounded more like a hockey skate careening to a halt just in front of the boards.

The first biopsy, back in Dr. Barkey's office, I was jaunty.

"You ain't got me, cancer. I got this."

For the second biopsy in Barkey's office, I was quietly confident, and a touch nervous.

My first biopsy in the University of Michigan clinic one week prior was a mix of scientific curiosity and terror.

This time, right from the outset, I was resigned. And edgy. And a little bit glum. As the adrenalin from my early skirmish with the doctor who chose the wrong work station wore off, I was also exhausted.

My Dad and Matt Ludgate chatted about biopsy procedures. As a proctologist, my Dad has plenty of experience with colorectal cancers. I was glad he was there. Ludgate was genuinely interested in my

Dad's work, which pleased me. Mort was genuinely interested in how Ludgate's day as a dermatology fellow shaped up. I enjoyed hearing Matt and Mort talking shop. While we may have lured my father there with the promise of a truly epic pastrami sandwich, he was intrigued by the science behind the procedure.

Matt finished the biopsies. Again, the tissues went into small, flat preservative-filled color-coded labeled trays. He began to stitch. I've been stitched a lot. After a burst elbow bursa on a mountainous descent during a bicycle road race pushed me over 200 stitches, I've given up count. Stitches are easy; a wee bit of pressure as the needle goes through the skin, a little tug, the sound of snip. Lather, rinse, repeat.

As I lay there, breathing through the stitches, I was thinking:

"Well, first biopsy, I freak out over the sound in my skull. Second go-round, I freak out because some poor doc wandered in to use a work station. If there's a third go-round, I'm either going to be all surfer dude, 'like, whoa, dude' and it'll be fine, or they'll have to give me some serious IV meds."

We'd promised Mort the best pastrami sandwich he'd had in years. I was hungry, as well. Panic, you realize, can do that to a man.

It is about two miles from the hospital to heaven. Zingerman's is heaven to the food-a-holic. Exotic foods, Jewish deli foods, extraordinary imported foods; all on display and many on sample, to boot. On a lovely sunny Tuesday at lunch time, we took our four inch thick sandwiches onto their deck. We left a trail of corned beef and pastrami and garlic pickle aroma in our wake. We took seats at the only open table.

The sandwiches were exceptional. The pickles were perfect. The iced tea was cold and crisp. Seated there, Mort and Cath compared notes about the procedure. They debated which freak-out of mine was more entertaining: the foul-mouthed carpet-bombing Cath was privy to, or the terrifying bombast with which I leveled an innocent physician. Happy to be outside, and that much closer to my problem's final solution, I eavesdropped on other conversations. My head swiveled around like a slow moving radar.

Click. Click. Click. It checked out the conversations of the day. Whoa, click, back up.

"I know that voice."

"What's that, Dave?" said Cath.

"Um, nothing. Did I say something?"

"Yes. Yes, you did. You said something about a voice."

"Yeah, right. Hang on a sec." I swiveled in my seat, snuck a peek in the direction of that voice, and swiveled back.

"Cath, look over my right shoulder. Isn't that the *Ca$h Cab* guy?"

She looked.

"You mean that guy with all those neck tats and the beads and stuff?"

"Yeah, him!"

"I don't know, I can't tell. The *Ca$h Cab* guy doesn't have all those tats and whatnot."

"Yeah, but he's always wearing t-necks and hoodies. Listen!"

We hear from behind us,

"Well, when I was doing stand-up, man, I always loved playing Ann Arbor. The crowds got my stuff, you know, and we always got food from here. Man, I miss Ann Arbor, but now that I've kinda broken out, I don't get back here enough."

"Oh my God," said Cath. "You're right. That's him; that's the *Ca$h Cab* guy."

Mort doesn't watch a lot of non-news or sports TV, except for Regis and Kelly. We explained the premise. A cab, driven by stand-up comedian Ben Bailey, picks up unsuspecting fares in midtown New York City. Once in the cab, a question and answer game show ensues. All of this plays out on TV, from the moment Ben Bailey picks up his fares to the moment he boots them out of his cab laden with their winnings. I tried not to shout out "AND THAT TRIGGERS a REEEEDD LIGHT CHAAAAAALLENGGGE!"

I started to get up.

Cath looked at me. "You're not going over there, are you?"

"Sure, why not? He's done eating. I'd never interrupt a man's corned beef sandwich. C'mon now, that'd be rude. I'm just gonna tell him I love his work and that's all, I promise."

Cath sighed. And shrugged.

"It's not like I can stop you. Go. Don't stay long."

I took the four steps over to his table. The *Ca$h Cab* guy was sitting there with two older women, the detritus of deli sandwiches in baskets before them.

"Hey, Ben Bailey! How are you?"

He looked up. A small smile started at the corners of his mouth. He nodded. He is very tall. Seated, he was nearly as tall as I am standing.

"Just wanted to say I love your stuff. Great show. Lots of fun."

My words came out in one big tumble.

"Oh, hey, that's cool. Thanks. Thanks a lot for stopping."

He paused and looked at my face. "Dude, what's up with…?"

He nodded towards my face, all scarred and tattoo-ed and dyed red and blue.

"Oh, that? Melanoma. They're trying to figure out how much skin needs to be removed. No big deal," I said.

Yes, I was lying. To me, it was a huge deal.

"Oh. Okay. Cool. Sounds like a big deal to me, but, okay, good luck with that, dude. And thanks for coming by."

Another day, another biopsy, my Dad, the best pastrami ever, and a brush with greatness.

I loved Ann Arbor that day.

Late that afternoon, Aaron asked about the day's procedure.

"Hey, how was Ann Arbor? How'd it go? Another couple meltdowns?"

"No, Mr. Aaron. Just one this time. And I got to meet Ben Bailey, the *Ca$h Cab* guy, that was cool, and there's half a Zingerman's sandwich for you, so there's that…"

"How many more of these you gotta do, Dad?"

"I wish I knew, kiddo. I hope this is the last one."

"Me, too, Dad. Now, about that sandwich?"

On Friday morning, our landline rang.

"Mr. Stanley. This is the U-M Melanoma Clinic. We have your lab results back. One of your new margins is clear. The other is not.

"We have several openings next week for your next biopsy. Do you have your calendar handy?"

Are We Done Yet?

Of course, I had my calendar handy. I always had my damn calendar handy when the landline rang. I was sick of laying on my right side in that tilt-a-chair with my left ear pointed to the heavens. I always felt like Hamlet's father the King, when Claudius poured poison into his ear.

I was sick of the sound of the double-edged scalpel ripping through my skin. Can you imagine the sound of three tween girl birthday parties when Justin Bieber walks in the room? Now, please mix in thirty college students anxious to start their weekend scraping chairs across the floor. For good measure, don't forget to throw in 20,000 crazy drunk South African soccer fans all blowing vuvuzelas as if they'd won the World Cup. The sound in my head was not as pleasant as all that. Plus, it was all inside my ear—a direct line to my auditory lobe.

It wasn't pain. I've had far worse pain. As a bike racer in my younger days, I crashed often and hard. Road rash from bike racing crashes hurts far worse. In the words of pro cycling manager Jonathon Vaughters, "Drive in a car going 30 miles an hour. Strip down to your underwear. Now, jump out." That's road rash, and at 1,200 highly disturbed nerve endings per square inch of skin, that's pain. My broken collarbone hurt far worse. If you've had a charley horse in the middle of the night, you've known greater pain. Dr. Ludgate's stellar technique and the power of local anesthesia skillfully applied insured that the biopsies were no more uncomfortable than a dental cleaning.

The frenzy was of my own invention. As the scalpel sliced shrilly through my skin, my ears sent the audio overload into my brain. My brain sent the message to the limbic system, the part of the brain that controls basic emotions and drives. As part of that system, my hippocampus, a set of deep ridges found at the base of each brain hemisphere's ventricle, did a dance of panic. Meanwhile, my amygdalae, two almond-shaped structures deep within the brain's temporal lobes, were overwhelmed with data and unable to stem the flood of neurotransmitters. Those transmitters told my adrenal glands that the body was in terrible danger and they better start pumping out epinephrine, also known as adrenaline: the "fight-or-flight" hormone. My body, after years of competitive sports, had become extremely good at cranking out the epinephrine. I could feel the panic rise, and I felt powerless to make it stop.

The morning of my third biopsy, Cath and I were accompanied by my mother. On the first trip to Ann Arbor, Cath and I were chatty. We could have been any couple commuting to work together. On the second trip, accompanied by my father, once we had decided that lunch at Zingerman's was on the schedule, the car fell silent.

On this trip, accompanied by my mother, and a much greater sense of my angst and anger, we were dead silent for the sixty-mile drive. I drove, my left hand draped over the top of the wheel and my right hand tucked under my right thigh, slumped down and leaning left in my seat. Morose and emotionally battered, I stared down the highway while NPR droned, barely audible in the car. Listing slightly to starboard in her seat, my wife dozed. Mom busied herself with a book in the backseat.

I was ready to be done. I was ready for the big surgery. Tell me the rules. Tell me what to expect. I can make myself comfortable. Not knowing, not being in control—I am not comfortable. I do not fly without Xanax. I am not afraid to fly. I am a bit claustrophobic, but in a plane, that's not my big issue. My big issue is that if I am not behind the controls, then I am not in control. I have always wrestled with the demon of control. Fortunately, my anxiety doesn't drive me to drink or eat or do recreational drugs.

It does drive me to exercise. My name is David L. Stanley and I have an exercise problem. I like to slay myself. I love to get on my bike and pedal, ride myself up to my redline and beyond, until I am so hypoxic my vision narrows into tiny black dots, just to see what's there, and then reel myself back in. I love to hit the weight room and lift until a swell of nausea hits my stomach and little bits of vomit spew up into my mouth and I have to choke it down until the set is over and I can get to the waste basket.

I find those feelings both therapeutic and cathartic. Admittedly, I have an endogenous endorphin addiction. By doctors' orders, all highly intense activity was forbidden. I could ride, and lift, but just hard enough to sweat. Exercise is the touchstone of my life. It's how I remind myself I am alive. Just hard enough to sweat was not hard enough. With that meditation removed from my life, I was a mental basket case.

We arrived. The first few times we exited the elevator, I was aghast at the state of the patients in the waiting area. Now, shuffling along, staring at my shoes, and feeling sorry for myself, these truly bad-ass survivors didn't even register. My case? My case was nothing compared to these warriors, but at that very moment, I was too busy with self-pity to pay attention.

I shuffled over to the check-in desks. I was too familiar with the routine. Say hi to the clerk, make a lame joke, hand her my ID cards, and hold out my wrist for the band, put out my other hand for the return of the cards, and head to the waiting area.

Once again, I had barely settled myself when my regular nurse came to fetch me. Perhaps it was my mien, perhaps it was the 70% humidity and 92 degree day, but she was less than perky. No matter. Showtime.

We walked back. She checked my wristband, flipped through my chart, and as she started to take my blood pressure, she looked at me.

"Not feeling yourself, are you, Mr. Stan, er, Dave?" she asked, remembering our conversation about being on a first name basis.

"Nope. Not so much. I mean, you're nice people here and all, but I'm just sick of all this. I just want to get this done. I am ready to move on to stage two.

"Oh, and don't forget I'm having that white…"

"That white coat hypertension? Yeah, that's pretty obvious."

She laughed.

I laughed, too. That would be my last laugh for the next hour and a half.

Dr. Ludgate was standing in the doorway, his entourage, larger than normal, trailing into the hall behind him. He heard our exchange.

"Dave, we're sorry to see you again, too, mate. I'd like to hit every margin on the first time, but you know that's not really possible, right? Look, I know this is not a comfortable procedure. But, it's not painful, is it? No, it's not."

I shook my head. "Nah, it doesn't hurt a bit. I'm just ready to move on."

Ludgate answered, "And even though you'd like to be done, I mean, geez, I'd like you to be done, too. But we both know this is going to give you the best possible outcome. We just cannot afford to have any pre-cancerous melanocytes left behind. End of story. If any get left behind, they will grow. I promise you that. And when they grow, well, as any surgeon will tell you, ask your Dad if you don't believe me, your best shot is always your first shot. After that, you have to work around stuff, or you need to dig even deeper. And that's more disfigurement. This time, after everything heals, you won't even be able to tell that you had surgery.

"The plastic surgery guys are that good, no worries. But that's with a clean field to work on. Second time around, all bets are off, mate."

"I know, I know. Just feeling beat up. A little pity party. I mean, I see those folks out in the lobby, that's some serious shit. My stuff, it's nothing. I know that. But today, I don't know why, I'm just dragging around."

"C'mon, let's get going," he said. "I'll do the anesthesia. Pathology gave me different guidelines for this last margin. It's going to be a wee bit bigger than the others, we're probably looking at a total field of about, oh, I'm guessing here, around 60 square centimeters. Seems big, I know, for a lesion that's only a centimeter, centimeter and a half across, doesn't it? We'll get everything this way, save you worry down the road, mate, and the next time you're in town, we can have a pint at the Red Hawk."

I lay down.

Dr. Matthew Ludgate went to work. A teeny pinprick, a slight burning sting, a numbness spreading across the side of my face, another poke, more burning, more numbness. Again and again and then, I felt Ludgate press on the side of my face.

"Feel that?" Dr. Ludgate asked.

"Nah, not really. Just a little pressure. You're good. Thanks for asking," I answered.

"I know you by now," he said. "I'm going to be working for a while. If you start to feel any discomfort at all, any, let me know. Without the epi, the anesthesia wears off faster. We don't want you to hurt. Don't be a hero. We have lots of anesthesia. Pints, quarts. Liters, even."

"Cool," I said. "Good to know."

"I know you hate this sound, but I need to get to work.

"See if you can fall asleep."

He chuckled.

"Yeah, right. Thanks for that thought," I said.

"Told you I know you pretty well by now, mate," he said.

And a thousand angry starving people scraped their knives across their plates inside my head.

Ludgate talked to me. About what, I cannot say. He was soothing, he gave me a play by play, he may well have told me ancient Maori stories of his childhood in New Zealand, but the young man did an amazing job of keeping me on the table without the need for IV sedation.

We were done.

Melanoma: It Started With a Freckle

He took another picture. I looked at the back of the camera. I now had a square within a square within a square tattooed and scarred into the side of my face. The area in front of my ear now bristled like infrequently shaved woman's leg, provided her leg hair was grey, black and white. The squares? An odd form of red and blue Russian nesting doll.

"Nice work, Doctor," I said. "Serious. You're good. Thank you."

I meant every word. His skills were that obvious. His stitching was perfect. The stitches were identical; tiny and neat with nary a pucker. Hollywood starlet facelift plastic surgery-worthy sutures. The red and blue dye was contained perfectly within each trough of a suture row. Very clean.

"Thank you, Mr. Stanley. Dave." he said. "I hope to not see you back here again. I am confident I won't. It's rare I can say this with such certainty, but you, sir, are going to be fine."

We shook hands. He turned and walked away. His entourage followed. It felt like the end of the classic Western *Shane*, when the hero walks away into the sunset.

A nurse led my wife and my mom back into the room.

"How'd it go?" asked mom.

"You were back there a long time," said Cath. "Way longer than the other times. This one was like twice as long. Everything go okay?"

"Twice as long? Huh, didn't seem that long."

I explained my existential crisis, how I pressed Ludgate into service as my therapist.

"Yeah, it went fine. Maybe I dozed off."

The nurse in the room snorted so hard that this time the Ovaltine did come out of her nose. I kid.

"Mrs. Stanley, I can assure you that your husband *did not* fall asleep," she said.

Cath raised an eyebrow and said, "Oooh, that I believe."

Mom sidled around to view the left side of my face. I watched her eyes get big as she took in the size of the latest margin. She frowned. She blinked. Frowned again.

"That's, um, pretty big, Dave," she said.

Cath moved over to look.

"Yep, that's a lot. At least, it's not moving towards your ear. I was worried about you losing your ear."

"Me, too, sweetie. I like my ear. And yep, it's big. Ludgate says it's like 50, 60 square centimeters. Big enough, anyway.

"Let's get the car and get out of here."

I was sick of Ann Arbor. I hated driving. I hated the hospital. I hated the cancer. I hated everything. Like an aura of evil, Hate radiated out from my body.

I felt fine. I wasn't sick. I was incubating a foreign body in my face that, without treatment, would kill me within two years. First, the cancer would disfigure me. More skin would be removed from my face. Some of the skin's underlayment would be removed, perhaps some bone, and the side of my face would cave in. The tumor would grow and swell, my vision destroyed as the cancer pushed my eye out of its socket. My sinuses would fill and the immense pressure would cause searing headaches.

In the other direction, the tumor would grow into my ear canal, putting pressure on my skull from within and my brain from without. Soon, like coarse grit sandpaper working against soft pine, the tumor would erode my face and all the organs in my neck. As the cancer traveled into my brain, it would divide and divide, destroying my brain cells as it made itself at home in my skull. If nothing else kills you first, the brain metastases will kill you.

Cancer: a parasitic beast, which cannot exist, so far as we know, outside of its host and yet, quite willing to kill its host in order to grow larger. So non-Darwinian.

It was a quiet car ride. It was the mirror image of the drive south to Ann Arbor. I drove. Cath dozed. Mom read. We went north.

Early that evening, Aaron came home from tennis practice. I was slumped in a chair, not reading the magazine I held in my hands.

"Hey!" he said.

"Hey, back," I said. "You seem happy."

"Yeah, practice was good. You shoulda seen me stripe my serve today."

Stripe: tennis lingo for hitting the lines. It's a good thing.

Aaron pantomimed a service motion in the den.

"Sooo… how'd it go?" he asked. "Panic? Terror? Fear and loathing?"

"No panic, kiddo. Just a little gloom. Kinda feeling sorry for myself. But, um, yeah, take a look. See what you think."

I turned so he could see the left side of my face.

"Hey, Dad?"

"Yeah?"

"That new line? That's, um, pretty big. Like really big."

"Yep."

"So, is that a good thing?"

"I hope so. Ludgate seemed to feel this was the last biopsy. He went out even further than pathology told him to, just to make sure. He's gotta be sick of seeing me. I know I'm tired of seeing him. They gotta get it all the first time, I know, but I am so ready to move on."

With a touch of fifteen year old boy awkwardness, my son reached over and patted me on the shoulder.

Several days later, the landline rang.

"Mr. Stanley. This is the U-M Melanoma Clinic. We have your lab results back. Your last margin is clear. The edges of your operative field are set."

"Next step, you'll need to have a consult with the surgeon. That's Dr. Moyer. He's a plastic surgeon who specializes in melanoma work.

"We'd like you to see him next week at his office in Livonia. We can set the appointment from here. Do you have your calendar handy?"

Part Three
The Intermission

In Which We Meet the Surgeon

"Was that the hospital?" asked Cath.

"Yep. Ludgate nailed the last margin. I'm done with all those biopsies. Done. Now it's time for the real surgery. Good Lord. Finally. I've, we've, been waiting for this all summer. I see the surgeon on Thursday. Eleven o'clock. His office is in Livonia. You wanna go with?"

"Really, David Stanley? Do I wanna go? Dumb question, dear. Very dumb question."

The 50-minute drive took us south from Flint on US-23, crosstown on I-96 east, and south again on I-275. The Detroit area traffic kept my mind occupied. As we exited the southbound freeway and drove across Haggerty Rd., we spotted the office complex. It was right next to a Bahama Breeze restaurant.

"Hey, look, babe! Bahama Breeze. We can grab some fish tacos for lunch after my appointment."

"Uh, yeah, great, dear. Not if you miss the entry to the doctor's office. That's your ADD talking. Let's just get you to your appointment first."

I missed the first entrance and pulled the car into the back parking lot. As I swung the car around, I saw a lovely dark green Porsche Boxster near the employee entrance. A Boxster with a bike rack on the rear deck.

"Must be the doctor's car," I said to Cath.

"You're thinking that's a good sign, aren't you?" she said.

"Could not be a better one," said the bike racing husband.

Walking into Moyer's office felt like walking into a jewelry store on Rodeo Drive. The lights were perfectly adjusted; dim, but not too. There were several perfectly artful displays for skin care products. Quiet jazz played. There were several women, perfectly coiffed and dressed, in the waiting room. They reminded me of mint condition Aston-Martin DB5s being dusted for fingerprints at a concours d'elegance; already in exquisite condition, and yearning for exquisite-er. *Town and Country* magazines were perfectly aligned on several coffee tables. A perfectly lovely coffee service sat in the corner. I was welcomed by a reception-ist who spoke no louder than a librarian. Clearly, my dermatologic surgeon also did a solid business in Botox and elective plastic surgery.

While Cath settled herself in the waiting area, I was ushered into Dr. Moyer's private office. A stack of charts sat on one corner of his desk. A silicone head-form sat on the other. He had a triptych of photographs on one wall; in them he was riding his time trial bicycle, running into a triathlon transition area, and exiting a lake in his wetsuit.

I had barely made a dent in the cushy chair in his office when the doctor strode in.

"Hi! I'm Dr. Moyer. Jeff Moyer. I'm taking over from Dr. Ludgate for your surgery. Melanoma aside, how are you?"

He sat down at his desk. He looked like a triathlete. Sandy hair, thin, graceful in his skin.

"Your case looks great. I've reviewed your chart, talked with Ludgate, everything looks really good. Getting to this lesion as soon as we did, we all feel very confident about your outcome. You should, too.

"Hey, Ludgate tells me you race bikes."

"Um, yeah. I started back in college, in the late seventies, and I just never quit. I was a soccer player at MSU, tore up my knee, started rid-ing for rehab, and sort of fell into the racing things. I race on the road, but I'm really a track racer at heart. I love racing the velodrome, flying around the bankings you pull a bunch of G's, you know? That's your Boxster out there with the bike rack, isn't it?"

"Sure is. Oh, man, I'd love to ride the velodrome," he said. "Looks like a riot, but seems kind of dangerous. If I crash? Dude, I need to think about my hands and wrists and everything. Bike legs in a tri are hairy enough for me. If I crash, then maybe that Boxster gets traded in for a pick-up, you know?"

"I know exactly what you mean," I said. "When I was 30, I started a new job in August. One week in, I crashed on the track in Detroit, endo-ed a couple of rotations, really stuck the landing hard, right on my shoulder, and broke my collarbone into four pieces. I had to wear Hawaiian shirts to work for the next three weeks. They were the only shirts I could get on over the brace without pain. In a financial services company. An old line company where casual Friday meant blazers and ties instead of suits. So, yeah. Crashing's bad. Hey, how'd you start do-ing tris anyway?"

"I ran track as an undergrad," Dr. Moyer said. "I did swim team in high school, just sort of segued into triathlon when I finished my resi-dency. A couple guys in our class did some tris, we went out for a ride,

I saw it was something I could get pretty good at, so I bought a bike. Then I got a wetsuit. Sound familiar?

"Hey, Dave, lemme show you something."

Moyer got up from his desk and walked to his closet. He rolled a beautiful Giant time trial bike in a luscious deep, rich blue, complete with disc wheel, out from the closet.

The perks of a hard-working physician, I thought. A Porsche and an $8,000 time trial bike. Nice.

"I have two more patients after you and then I leave for Chicago. Triathlon this weekend."

He leaned the bike against his office wall and walked to his desk. He picked up the head form and a marker.

"C'mon, let's go into an exam room and I'll give you an idea of what's going to happen."

I sensed Dr. Moyer had removed his cycling helmet and donned his doctor hat.

He held the head-form in the crux of his arm. As we entered the exam room, he inked a dot on the spot of my lesion, just in front of the left ear's tragus. I hopped up on the exam table. Head-form under his arm, Moyer sat down on a rolling chair next to me.

He drew a square's worth of dotted lines around the dot. It was a fair approximation of the sutures on the side of my face.

"Here are the margins that Dr. Ludgate determined. I like to go out a bit further at every margin, maybe two, three millimeters or so. I'll determine that in a few minutes, when I do your work-up. That gives us even more margin for error. With cancer cells you never know, so I'll remove everything, down as far as I need to. Everything needs to be cleaned out. Skin, underlying soft tissue, all of it comes out. The muscles stay, because we got to this lesion early.

"I leave the nerves, as much as possible. Nerves, you know, they don't like to grow back, they don't regenerate well, and I want you to have good sensation in your cheek. And you know, if the nerves get nicked, you might lose some muscular control, like you had a small stroke. We don't want that. Bad for you, bad for your looks, bad for my rep."

He laughed. I joined in. I got it. I didn't want that either. I wanted normal back.

"Now, there are also several small arteries, I'll leave all them in place, too. Capillaries, we don't care about them, they'll regenerate. But in general, this is a very careful, very thorough dissection.

"Look, I say this to all my cancer patients, you see those other patients out there, the facelifts, and nose jobs, I like doing that work, but this, this kind of work…"

He nodded at me.

"This kind of work is why I'm a doctor.

"Don't get me wrong, the Botox does pay the bills."

He shrugged, laughed, and waved towards his bike.

"Wrinkles do have their advantages, don't they?" I said.

"Indeed. Yes, indeed," he answered.

Dr. Moyer put the head form on the workspace beside him. He drew a solid line. It started near the head-form's temple, went straight across to the top of the ear, turned 90 degrees due south, right down to the ear lobe at bottom, and then wrapped it up and behind the ear. He had drawn a square root symbol, in mirror image.

"That's about where your scar line will be. I'll pull everything up to that line. You'll have some staples, and quite a few stitches."

He walked over to my chair. He had a small lens in one hand.

"Let me see what we have here. Hold still, wouldja?"

Again, just as with Barkey, and Ludgate, I had a physician breathing in my ear.

His hands were on the side of my face. He palpated along my outermost sutures. It felt as if he was drumming his fingers, in slow motion, along the desk that was my face. I felt a few gentle pinches.

"I think you'll be okay. No graft," he murmured. "I can't really tell until we get into the OR, but I suspect you won't need a graft. For an old guy, heh-heh, your skin seems elastic enough. Still, you never know. If I need a graft I'll pull it from the front of your shoulder. That's the best spot for a face. It'll match up to your complexion nicely—no one will ever know.

"I am pretty good at this plastics stuff."

I laughed.

"I never doubted..."

"Well, I have done this before," he said. "I did an ENT residency, did ENT for a few years, then I did a plastics and reconstruction post-doc. I do as much of the head and neck cases for the melanoma clinic as I can."

"So you have some skills. Nice. What about my post-op?" I asked.

"Right. Well, we'll send you home right away. Not a high risk of infection, there's no real post-op care needed. You'll be a lot more comfortable at home. I'll write some pain meds, but most of my patients say it's pretty low level pain, discomfort really. You've had worse from crashes, I promise. This is nothing compared to your broken collarbone. I know you've had way worse from road rash, I guarantee it. Ice packs help a lot. Keeps the swelling down, helps the pain."

Dr. Moyer continued.

Melanoma: It Started With a Freckle

"You want a good result, right? Then, here's what you have to do. One, don't let your head get below your chest for the first five days. Do *not* bend over. Just don't. If you can't get your wife to get something for you, you could squat down, I guess, but you really need to keep your head up to avoid swelling. I use a pressure bandage but still… Rule Number One: No Bending Over. Got it?"

I nodded.

"Yes, sir."

I got it.

"Good. Two: do not twist your neck for the first three days. We do not want any torque on your head or neck. You need to look to the side, turn at the waist. There's nothing over there, anyway. We cannot have anything, I mean anything, pull on your stitches. You pull on those stitches, you'll gap the incision, it'll heal that way, and then I'll need to do a scar revision. I hate doing scar revisions. Don't do that to me. No twisting."

He read my mind, one athlete to another.

"Look, I get it," he said. "Your big concern is when you can start training again. In your mind, you're already healed. No BS, now. This is major surgery. You'll be out for 4 hours. Minimum. Major procedure.

"When you get home, you do nothing. Nothing. No driving, for five days. Hear me? Just because I'm sending you home, don't get the idea that this is no big deal. You're going to be under for half the day. This is a big deal. There is a lot of trauma involved in this surgery. Just like a hard training block, your body needs time to recover.

"For sure, don't think of training for two weeks. Minimum. Don't even think about riding the trainer. Anyway, I don't think you'll feel like it. It's a lot of anesthesia. You'll probably spend the first three, four days sleeping, but I'm telling you this anyway. You can go for short walks, go out and get a little air, ten minutes, tops.

"No training until I say so. I'll see you one week after the surgery and we'll sort it out then. Plan on missing two weeks of work, okay?

"The sooner we do this, the better. The hospital will call you tomorrow to set the OR date.

"Now, get outta here. Two more patients. I got a race in Chicago to get to."

Over orders of fish tacos and iced tea, Cath and I talked about the plan.

"I want to do this ASAP, Cath. I mean, if we can do this Monday, I'm for it. I just want this over."

"I get that, honey, but what about work?" Cath continued, "Don't you want to go to work for a week, meet your classes, train up your kids, get everything ready for your sub, and *then* have the surgery? Doesn't that seem like a good plan?

"You've been under all this stress all summer. I watch you, you know. Seems like it'd be a good stress reliever to go to work for a few days, hang out with your work peeps, and then have the surgery. I mean, it's up to you, but I think you should consider going to work first."

I thought for a few moments. Cath was right. Of course, she was right. That was the correct plan. I like correct plans.

"Okay. Done. I'll schedule the surgery for the Monday after Labor Day week."

The phone rang Friday morning.

"Mr. Stanley. This is the U-M Melanoma Clinic. We understand your pre-op meeting with Dr. Moyer yesterday went well. He'd like us to go ahead and schedule your surgery so if you have…"

I interrupted.

"Right. I want to have the surgery the Monday after Labor Day week. We're coming down from Flint so can we do maybe 8 am so we don't have to get up at 5 to get there on time, what with rush hour traffic and all?"

"Well, Mr. Stanley. We don't do an 8 o'clock. We can make it for 9, though, if that's okay?"

"Nine is great. I've got it down."

"Okay, Mr. Stanley. You'll go to the regular melanoma clinic first for check in, and then they'll walk you to the OR for surgery check-in. You'll need a driver for the ride home. You're going to receive a packet from us in the mail in a day or two. Make sure you fill it out before you arrive and, please, make sure you follow the pre-op directions quite closely. If you don't, they won't be able to do your surgery as planned.

"Later this week, you'll get a phone call from one our clinic nurses to answer any questions, double check that you understand the pre-op instructions. Do you have any questions? No? Then we'll see you at check-in on Monday.

"Try and relax, Mr. Stanley. It's hard, I know. You notice I said try?"

Exit, Stage Right Even:
The Staff Meeting

"'Relax', she says. Not bloody likely," I thought.

I have a B.Sc. in zoology from Michigan State. I studied physics, chemistry, biology, and anatomy. I teach students who are often driven to do research just to see if they can trip me up with a question in class. Nothing pleases my students more than a lengthy digression on a big question that involved a lot of classroom discussion. They never notice that I always manage to lead their question back to my curriculum. But I digress.

I'm a science nerd. I browse Wikipedia and PLOS: the Public Library of Science. I subscribe to more than a handful of science dork websites and email lists. Even before my initial diagnosis, I was scientifically intrigued by melanoma. One, I have been a huge Bob Marley fan since college. The idea that a small tumor on Marley's right large toe could spread to his brain astounded me. Marley, it was discovered much later, had acral melanoma: a rare form found on the palms of hands, the soles of feet, and around the large toe. It is not linked to UV exposure. Two, I teach a large unit on genetics to my biology students. DNA mutations have always played a major role in the rules of engagement for my students. It is those mutations, cause by UV over-exposure that had me in this spot.

In the world of cancer treatment, melanoma can be a real SOB to treat. Here's why.

Because melanocytes are related to neural germ cells, melanoma is prone to travel to the brain and set up their tumor shop inside one's cranium. This can happen with even barely noticeable lesions. UV radiation, especially as a teen and young adult, will cause DNA mutations that create the conditions for melanoma in later life. Most melanomas have little genetic basis. About 8% of people newly diagnosed with melanoma have a first-degree relative with melanoma. About 1–2% have two or more close relatives with melanoma. One study shows that changes in the *CDKN2A* (*p16*) gene cause some melanomas to run in certain families. But in the main, it's the UV exposure.

In the DNA molecule, remember that cytosine (C) bonds with guanine (G), and that adenine (A) bonds with thymine (T). You have about three billion pairs of C–G and A–T in each strand of your DNA. Each base pair is roughly 2–3 angstroms from the next pair down the helix. An angstrom is 1×10^{-10} of a meter. That's one ten billionth of a meter. In other words, very small, far smaller than our brains can grasp easily.

With some exceptions (sex cells, e.g.), each of your cells contains a complete complement of your DNA. A typical cuboidal hepatocyte (liver cell) is 200,000 angstroms on the edge. Wadded up inside that cell, inside of every cell in your body, in its nucleus, is a ball of DNA 60,000 angstroms across. That's small beyond normal human belief.

You can't see it with the unaided eye. You can't see one hepatocyte either. The human eye, a darn fine eye by the way, is capable of resolving things as small as 1,000,000 angstroms across. That's one-tenth of one millimeter. In other words, a young person with good near vision could almost see a Rubik's cube made from hepatocytes.

Should you manage to extract your DNA strand in its entirety from a cell and stretch it out, it would be roughly two meters long. Should you manage to extract all the DNA from the ten trillion cells in your body and stretch them end to end, your DNA would make about 1500 roundtrips to the moon.

That's a lot of trips. It is also a lot of opportunity for things to go wrong. Too much exposure to UV radiation messes with this arrangement. Thirty years in the sunshine created far too many T–T thymine pairs, known as dimers, in my skin's DNA. These mutations were first repaired by my body, but too much sun, over too many years, overwhelmed my cellular repair mechanisms. My T–T pairings started to copy each other, as DNA pair bonds are instructed to do. What happened when I accumulated enough thymine dimers in the right location of my double helix? Melanoma.

Surgery, when I was diagnosed, was the only option. Even today, in late 2015, only a handful of chemotherapy agents have been approved, and they do not work across the board.

Melanoma, don't forget, is an exceptionally sneaky rat bastard. Many types of melanoma utilize a cloaking device of near-Romulan Warbird proportions. These melanoma cells are covered with a protein coat as a form of camouflage. This protein is one which is produced in a normal, healthy body. The body does not recognize this protein coat as being that of an intruder. Ergo, the body's immune system does not know to spring into action. To date, an immune therapy drug to counteract that cancerous cloaking device has been helpful in only 20–30% of patients.

Surgery, then, it is.

I returned to work. Teachers have plenty of pre-season training camp meetings. Our staff, 120 strong, breakfasted together in the school cafeteria on the opening day of training camp. Seated with my cronies, my posse, my partners in crime, I explained the Russian nesting dolls of stitchery on the side of my face. I told the story of "How I Spent My Summer" to six of my closest friends. I explained the upcoming procedure, my timeline, and the expected outcome. I gave them their marching orders; to explain my situation to our colleagues so that I was spared the rehash of the story.

We had a speaker in the morning. A short, pudgy, grey-haired white man in an ill-fitting suit, he was the epitome of a life-long mid-level bureaucrat. He spoke to the entire staff in the auditorium about economic developments in our school district's county. He stood in front of PowerPoint slides which were cut and pasted in from a governmental white paper written by people just like him.

He was terrible. Ferris Bueller's *"Anyone? Anyone? The tariff bill? The Hawley-Smoot Tariff Act? Which, anyone? Raised or lowered?… raised tariffs,"* would have been an improvement. We passed the hour texting each other, hands shielding the light of our phone screens like a bunch of our students. I received dozens of texts wishing me well. It was nice. It also made it impossible to get my surgery off of my mind.

At the end of the day, we gathered in the kiva for a few small presentations from colleagues and a wrap-up. Many of my colleagues are excellent presenters but I was too exhausted to listen. My eyes struggled to stay open. I felt as drained as if I'd done a 100-mile bike ride instead of merely sitting on my rear for seven hours. Foolishly, I sat there and re-read my friends' supportive texts on my phone. I felt my heart rate speed up. I put my phone in my pocket. My mind sped up.

Mentally, I fast-forwarded two weeks, to that Monday morning when I would become pharmaceutically unconscious, paralyzed, intubated, and then, operated upon for perhaps five hours while my wife sat in a waiting room. My heart rate did not slow down.

I half-closed my eyes. I breathed in and out. I tried to match my breath to a slow count of One…Two…Three…Four… Crap. Not at all useful.

I tried rational thought.

"This is surgery. You worked in an OR. These folks are expert. You are far more likely to be in a car accident on the way to the hospital than you are to have a bad surgical experience. All of your doctors have stressed how confident they are in this procedure."

My heart rate did not slow down. My breathing became shallow and rapid. I recognized the symptoms. This was the beginning of a panic attack. I had the vaguest of sensations that I was watching myself panic.

Quietly and smoothly, I thought, I got up from the conference table. Suavely, I headed to the door. A bathroom break, everyone would think. Once in the hall, I pulled out my phone, dialed Cath, and, shit, she was out and her cell phone went straight to voicemail. Heart racing, my mind keeping right up, I dashed down the hall to men's room. I splashed cold water on my face. Water dripping down my chin and off my nose, I stared at my face in the mirror.

Déjà vu.

"I've done this before," I said to my reflection. "I've heard that presentation before. I felt the panic attack on its way. I got up and left the room before. I called Cath. I washed my face."

I replayed the last few minutes, having a difficult time separating reality from my subconscious.

As I cupped my hands under the spigot, I let the cold water run over my face and into my mouth. I washed my face again. I dried it. I stood up and looked into the mirror. An ashen damp face stared back at me. I made the decision to go and sit in the stairwell and look out the window for a few minutes. Out of body déjà vu aside, I was now certain I was at work.

As I approached the stairwell, my colleagues BP and Amy Jo were standing there in wait.

"What was that all about?" asked BP.

"Wha? I dunno, I just, just needed to go to the bathroom, I guess," I said.

"Really?" said Amy Jo. "You get up in the middle of Derek's presentation, he's starting to answer a question, you dash out of there like a madman. Hell, you bashed into a chair on your way out."

"No, I didn't, I…I just… um," I stammered.

Not as suave as I thought.

BP stood right in front of me. He grabbed me by the upper arms.

"Dude, you all right?" he asked.

I don't recall a man ever looking that deeply into my eyes before.

"Seriously," said Amy Jo. "I mean, what the hell? You feel okay? You're as white as Hamlet's ghost. If you were one of my kids, I'd say you just had a bad dream."

BP let go of my arms.

Melanoma: It Started With a Freckle

I explained, as best I could, the panic attack, the déjà vu, the out of body experience. They nodded at me.

Amy Jo stepped in front of me. In her best teacher voice she said, "You go home. We got this. You need to get the hell outta here. Take the back roads. Listen to some quiet music in the car. Roll down the windows. Breathe. Now. Go. Namaste."

BP joined in.

"I'll talk to the chief. Want me to leave out all that altered states of consciousness crap and just tell him you don't feel well?"

Opening Day of school was six days later. I decided to address my situation, first thing, with every class. No elephants in the room. I'd been a teacher and coach at Holly High School for six years. I was part of the crew. I'd had some of the older students before. Many of the freshmen knew of me, either by reputation or via siblings. My kids needed to know the plan for the first few weeks of school. I'd be their teacher for a week. I had carefully selected one substitute for the next two weeks. The lessons he'd teach were my lessons. After two weeks with the sub, I would return.

My first day's lesson plan was simple. I'd tell the kids I had cancer. I'd show them my stitches. I would explain the biopsy procedure. I'd tell them I met the *Ca$h Cab* guy. I would give them the low-down on my surgery and expected recovery. I would put questions out to them about their cancer experiences. We would have a few warm and fuzzy moments.

I put together a PowerPoint slide show on melanoma: why it's so dangerous, the genetics and mutation, how to recognize the A-B-C-D-Es of the disease, the importance of sunscreen; I'd urge them to remind their parents to get weird moles and skin things checked. I used a few Bob Marley songs for the soundtrack.

I'm a science teacher. Everything's a lesson.

Part Four
The Main Symphony

Amped Up in Pre-Op

My panic attack, night terrors, and general tumult aside, the first week of school was great. I showed the kids my "tattoos." I taught my melanoma lesson. We discussed the high likelihood that I would be a melanoma survivor. We discussed cancer. Every kid, in every class, of course, had been touched by cancer. Day Two, we moved right into "school." The kids who were bound to act like little twits acted like little twits. The kids who were just cruising through with a gentleman's (or lady's) C, began their cruise. The kids gunning for As were locked and loaded. It was school. Business as usual.

"I can't open my locker."

"Where is Mrs. Tomlinson's room?"

"What lunch period do we have?"

"When's our first test?"

"I hate that kid. I can't sit next to him."

"Do we haveta know this? Really?"

It was good for my psyche to be engaged with my students again. For big chunks of the day, I did not think about surgery, or cancer, or the possibility of a bad outcome. The kids were great. The best way to influence kids is to model the behavior you wish to see. I behaved as if this was no big deal, and so did my students. Older students who heard the news stopped by to wish me the best. My colleagues in the beige pod behaved as if nothing was amiss. At this point, pre-surgery, they were more interested in who my substitute might be and if they'd be needed to ride herd on my kids.

Once the school week was over, and Cath and I were home for the weekend, things became a wee bit pear shaped. It was stressful. We did not have an elephant in the room. We talked so much that the elephant became bored and left the room. We did the best we could to remind ourselves of all the positives: early detection of the original lesion, cleanly delineated margins, a very competent surgeon, outpatient surgery, the extremely low chances of a bad anesthesia experience, U-M's outstanding track record with melanoma. We're both science people. We get it.

Didn't matter; two very nervous people were southbound in the car on the way from Flint, Michigan to Ann Arbor on that Monday morning.

I am not normally a nervous person. I am, however, highly energetic. When I get excited about something, I drag people along with me. People end up joining rugby teams, or jumping out of planes, or doing shots of Jack Daniels and then getting up at 6:00 am to get the first chairlift up the hill on a powder skiing day. The other side of that energy, as Anakin Skywalker would agree, is that energy can be shifted with a just a teeny nudge in the right place, into a very bad place.

Cath knows this. Her plan? Leave early on Monday morning, well before the traffic, and go for a calming, spirit-soothing walk in one of Ann Arbor's beautiful parks along the Huron River. Genius. Normally, Flint to A² is a sixty minute drive. We were expected at the hospital at 8:50 for our 9:00 am admit.

We hit the road at 6:15. We had quiet classical music, *Mozart in the Morning,* playing on the CD. I made a conscious effort to stay in the right hand lane and travel 70 mph. All was going according to plan until we hit a construction zone near the small town of Brighton forty minutes down the road. We were stopped dead. Under the best of circumstances, I am not good at being stuck in traffic.

This morning was not the best of circumstances. In this pre-smart-phone GPS era, it was not possible to leave the highway for an alternative route. It took all of Cath's considerable psychiatric nursing skills to keep me under control as we sat motionless and unaware of the problem up ahead. We were dead in the water amidst of a sea of anxious motorists.

After ten minutes, traffic began to move smoothly again. A line of sand and gravel trucks, which needed to get across to the center median for concrete repair work, had shut down traffic whilst they got themselves into position, dumped their loads, and then retreated back onto the southbound access lane.

I wish I had been wearing my heart rate monitor at that moment. I believe I hit a new peak heart rate during those five minutes.

Ann Arbor, as the name implies, is a beautiful town. Also known as Tree Town, and A², Ann Arbor features loads of greenscaping, and parks everywhere. Cath directed me to Gallup Park. We arrived at 7:30 am, just as the sun was fully risen on an early September morning. The morning dawned misty and cool. A few runners darted about. Moms and dads pushing strollers were out in force. The odd rollerblader or two put in appearances. Ten minutes from the hospital, we had an hour to walk the exercise path, sit at picnic table, hold hands, and talk calmly and quietly with each other.

In a fashion, sitting there at the table on a cool, foggy morning, it felt like a stage of a honeymoon. Once the initial crazy wild sex of the honeymoon night fades for a few moments, you lay there with each other and gaze at each other. You are dumbfounded at how much you love this person, and you are equally dumbfounded that this person loves you that much right back.

There we sat, holding hands and talking, and feeling like that. My mouth was very dry. I was having difficulty forming words. I had been NPO (nil per os—nothing by mouth) since midnight. No food, no water, no ice. I was also pretty damn nervous. I was not terrified, ready to out-run a charging bear scared. I was a steady thrumming in the background, overstimulated amygdala "right on the edge of crazy" kind of scared.

Adrenalin, it dries you out.

"Hey, Cath. You got any mints? I'm really dry."

You know you're NPO. No mints."

"Oh. Right. I knew that. Thanks. How about some gum?"

"Gum? Yeah, gum's probably fine. Sure, here."

I unwrapped. I chewed. Moisture restored. Verbal dexterity restored, the crisis was averted.

It was time. Our visit to the park was a perfect moment. I felt calm. We parked the car and found our way to check-in. It was 8:45 am as we approached the check-in desk in the surgery waiting area.

I handed my ID cards to the clerk.

Hands flying, doing an excellent Barney Fife impression, she squawked, "Where have you been? We've been trying to get ahold of you all morning. This is making things very complicated."

Being faced with a woman who appeared to be right on the edge of a meltdown did not do much for my emotional state. I was in a state: either I would rip this woman's head from her neck or I would break down in tears. Cath stepped up.

"We were told to be here at 8:50. It's 8:45. We are on time. And I can't imagine that you tried very hard to reach us. My husband and I both have phones, and neither phone rang this morning."

"We had a no-show," she dithered, "and we needed to fill that slot to keep everything moving smoothly for everyone. Well, you finally got here and that's good."

"Again, we were on time. Early, in fact," said Cath.

David L. Stanley

"And since all your slots were filled before the no-show, I don't see how our being early could possibly have disrupted your patient flow. And last, my husband is very anxious. He is facing a very long procedure and your, whatever this handwaving is about, is *really* not helping his mental state.

"Where do we go, now that check-in is complete?"

Anxious? Yes, I was very anxious. Just watching this frantic little woman had kicked my fight or flight reflex into top gear.

A few moments after we sat down, a nurse came for me. A calm, pleasant, typical U-M melanoma clinic nurse.

"I'll take you back," she said, looking at me, "and then once he's changed into a gown, and I've got the pre-op work going, I'll call up here for you, Mrs. Stanley."

We walked down the hall. Me on the right side, her on the left side of the hall. In a gentle voice, she asked questions. I answered as best I could.

"You're here for a…?" she asked.

"The last part of my square procedure," I finished her sentence.

"Right. And where are they working to..?"

As she said this, she happened to glance over at me.

"Oh. Right. Never mind, then."

I was led to a gurney inside the pre-op area. She handed me a gown, dark blue bootie socks with maize block Ms across the insteps, and a hairnet. I was told to remove all my clothes, including my drawers, all my jewelry, and don the hospital wear. She pulled the curtain around my gurney, with a metallic rush and rattle of curtain rings over curtain rods. I removed my shoes. I re-tied my shoes before I placed them in the bag; left shoe to the left and right shoe to the right. I undressed as slowly as possible. I was anxious to get on with the show and simultaneously, I wanted to freeze time. I re-buttoned my polo shirt up to the neck and re-zipped the fly on my Bermuda shorts. I folded my clothes with a precision which outpaced any seen on laundry day, and placed everything in the bag which Cath would receive. I stuck my head out of my curtained-off cubicle.

"I'm ready."

I sat down on the edge of the gurney. The linens were covered with hundreds of tiny block Ms.

A plastic thermometer probe went under my tongue. A blood pressure cuff went around my arm. A small plastic device, a pulse oximeter that would measure oxygen saturation in my blood, went over the end of my finger. The nurse's fingers palpated for my pulse. Cath walked into the cubby. Pulse was normal. Temperature was normal.

I noticed the pre-op area was huge. There were perhaps five dozen gurneys back there.

"Big as a hockey rink," I noticed.

Heart rate was acceptable. I'm usually around 52–56. This morning, I was in the mid-70s. The nurse made notes.

Not only was the pre-op area huge, it was bustling. It seemed as if each patient gurney had three or four people tending to it. It was pretty clear to me that this was SOP. No one was nervous. No one rushed about. Unlike the wacky check-in lady, these were pros being pro.

I started to calm down after the check-in fiasco. I heard the monitor's beepbeepbeepbeepbeepbeep slow down to beepbeep beepbeep beepbeep. I focused on the sound. I tried to sync my breathing with the beeping. It worked. I slowed everything down a bit more beep beep beep beep   beep beep.

Blood pressure? Acceptable.

"Okay, I can do this," I thought.

Cath sat quietly as the nurse started running through a few questions.

"Are you in any pain right now? Did you urinate this morning? Do you feel the need now? When did you last have a bowel movement? When did you last have anything to eat or drink?"

"Well, I guess, dinner, you know, and then I had some iced tea after that, so I don't know, probably around ten o'clock last night. They told me I was NPO so…"

"That's good. You can't have anything in your stomach during surgery. It can be very dangerous. They don't even like you to have much saliva, if you can help it. You might vomit it up, and then it could end up in your lungs or trachea. That's bad news, when that happens."

"Saliva? Well, I had a really dry mouth an hour ago, so I chewed some gum," I said.

"Gum?"

Her jaw dropped.

"Yeah, just for a few minutes. It was sugar free so I spit it out pretty fast. Ten minutes, tops," I said.

She blinked.

"I'm not sure about that gum. No mints, I know. This could be a problem. I need to check with anesthesia right away. I hope they don't need to reschedule your surgery. I'll be right back. There's the head of anesthesia."

BEEPBEEPBEEPBEEPBEEPBEEP!!!!!!!

The thought of putting this off any longer over a piece of gum was sending me over the edge. The beeps sounded like a staccato blast coming from Miles Davis's trumpet. My heart rate was in triple digits.

David L. Stanley

My BP was no longer acceptable. My hands were gripping the safety rail so tightly that my hands were as white as frostbite. My feet were kicking back and forth like an angry toddler. I was bouncing up and down on the gurney.

I watched my nurse talking to a kid who looked like he'd be more at home on a surfboard than being the chief of anesthesia in a University hospital. He looked at me, and back at the nurse. I suspect I looked as near to panic as I felt. He bent low to talk with her. I couldn't see his mouth, couldn't hear a word.

He hustled over.

"Oi, mate. I'm the chief of anesthesia in here today," he said in a perfect Melbournian accent. "Tell me mate, what'd you do this morning?"

The words came out in a rush. Nothing to eat or drink since 10 pm. The visit to the park. The dry mouth. The sugar-free gum which lost its flavor quickly and I spit out after ten minutes. My face felt hot and sweaty. My shoulders were up around my ears. The monitors were keeping an allegro beat.

"So the gum was around 8:00, you think? Right-o, it's 9:30, sugar free doesn't generate much saliva production. We're good, I think, mate. That was a close one. We'll be fine."

Looking at the nurse, he said, "Make sure that's in the chart, and I'll sign it off. The room needs to know."

He looked up the monitors. He looked at me. He took my arm and felt for my pulse. He turned my hand palm down.

"You've got great veins, mate. Your IV will go in, no worries. I've got one more patient to see to, I'll be back in a minute, and then we'll get you started. Try to take a few deep breaths, calm down a bit. I'm not sending you home. We're gonna do this today. You'll be apples. Right-o, breathe now, would you? Right. Back in a second."

I was teetering on the edge of panic. I had psyched myself up for surgery TODAY. The thought that chewing a piece of gum had nearly sent me home, to return a few days later, had methatclose to a full-on panic attack.

I lay back on the gurney. I breathed. In through the mouth and out through the nose, in through the mouth and out through the nose. I tried to home in on the buzz of the overhead lights. I tried to focus on a spot above and between my eyes. I tried to slow down the beeping behind my head on the monitor screens. I failed.

My fingers were drumming on the gurney, keeping rhythm to an unheard Santana song.

The anesthesiologist returned and grasped my hand, and said "Hi, I'm back," in a gentle voice.

100

I sat stark upright in bed.

"Lay back, mate," he said.

"No. I do better when I can supervise. I like to know what's going on."

He nodded. He'd seen this before.

"I'm going to start your IV now," he said.

I've had plenty of IVs. A big hollow needle surrounded by a Teflon tube is slid into a vein in the back of the hand. The needle is backed out. This leaves the tube behind and the drip gets hooked up. No pain. Easy.

He reached into an anesthesia tool belt he was wearing. He took out a syringe the size of a diabetic's dose of insulin.

He slid it into the back of my hand.

"WHAT THE HELL IS THAT?"

Heads turned all around my end of the pre-op area.

"Shh, mate. Quiet down. You're scaring people. Really. Stop it. Right now. Okay, good. It's some Novocain. We like to inject a little into the IV site. It makes people more comfortable when the IV goes in. Okay?"

I was now in full-on panic mode.

"I've had lots of IVs. I've never seen that before. I told you I need to know what is going on."

I was spitting words like an Eminem rap.

"I gotta tell ya," I went on, "I'm about ready to just get up and run right the hell out of here. This morning has just been totally fucked: the traffic jam, and that batshit crazy lady at check-in, and the gum, and I'm fucking scared to death anyway cause I'm gonna be in there for I don't know how long and my wife'll just be sitting there and I don't know how I'm even managing to stay here in this gurney cause I wanna get up and run right down that hall."

I was hyperventilating. The monitors were one long beeping beep. I was soaking wet. Most likely, my underarms smelled like fetid pools.

I stopped to catch my breath.

The IV was in. This Aussie, he was good.

"Mr. Stanley, I can help you with that. I want to inject a little medicine into your IV. It'll take the edge off. This stuff is good. You'll feel better, right away, I promise. Is that okay?"

"Anything is better than the way I feel right now, so if you promise it'll work fast, yeah, go."

He drew another small syringe from his belt kit, uncapped it, and slid the needle into the extra valve in my IV. Before he even withdrew the needle, the meds started to work.

My breathing slowed. My brain stopped racing. I looked at the anesthesiologist.

"Wow. Holy crap. Dude, that stuff's amazing."

"It hasn't even really kicked in yet. Give it a second."

Within moments, I was totally relaxed. I felt like I'd just had my second glass of chilled Gewürztraminer on the deck on a lovely Friday evening.

I sat up and looked at the doctor.

"Hey! I like this. Man, I want to feel like this all the time. So, what part of Melbourne you from? I have some friends over there. What brought you to the States?"

I was babbling, but I was babbling, thanks to modern pharmacology and a smooth Aussie anesthesiologist, in a most reasonable way.

"Mrs. Stanley," he said to Cath, "why don't you give your husband a hug and a kiss and we'll get started while this stuff is working so well. He's going to be fine, but I really do need to get him to the OR. Dr. Moyer and his crew are waiting."

My wife and I hugged and kissed.

Cath said, "I'll see you in a few. Lay back, honey. They can't move you while you're sitting up."

Cath, the nurse, and the doctor all looked at each other, shocked, I suspect, at the sudden rate of psychological turnaround.

"I'll take him myself," the doctor said.

I laid back and we rolled down the hall.

"If this stuff works so well, why didn't you give it to me sooner?" I asked.

"Well, Mr. Stanley, I didn't expect that you'd freak out quite that badly. That was quite a performance, mate."

"Um, yeah. About that, I was a little surprised, too," I said.

"We're here."

The gurney was next to the surgical table. The room was calm. The lights seemed pink. There were four or five people, male and female, in the room. They were gloved, gowned and masked, but I sensed they were smiling under the masks. Their eyes were crinkly, in a good way. Someone, a female, asked me to scoot over. I scooted.

The anesthesiologist, my new best friend, was now masked. He was standing by my head with a gas mask in his hand. He was looking down at me. I got the distinct impression he was chuckling under his mask. He placed the mask gently over my face.

"There's a lot of oxygen in this mask, mate. Lots. And you need some extra oxygen right now, so take some deep breaths, right, deep breaths… there you go…"

A little fib, it wasn't just oxygen in that mask.

Cath Waits

14

At this point, I assume the team got to work. Being under anesthesia, intubated, and with an IV pushing paralyzing medications through my circulatory system, I can only guess. Cath had plenty of time to kill. Alone.

Normally, my parents would have accompanied her. Cath's family is from Saint Louis, Missouri, and that is quite a trek to sit in a waiting room with their daughter. Being retired, my parents have plenty of time on their hands and I am their eldest son. However, my Dad had just undergone a stay in the hospital. A bad reaction to ibuprofen had thrown his 75-year-old kidneys for a loop. Mom and Dad needed to stick close to home. We had several friends volunteer to sit with Cath. As my surgery was not expected to be "life threatening" (indeed, it was life-saving), we asked them not to take time away from work.

Cath is a nurse. In fact, she was a nurse in a University of Michigan clinic which used these same surgical suites. Cath had often walked with patients back into pre-op, and escorted them into the surgical suites. Having recently stepped into a new position, she still had plenty of work friends in the building. She decided against visiting around the hospital and made her way into the waiting area.

Cath didn't last long in the waiting area. If you have ever spent much time in a surgical waiting lounge, you know there is nothing restful about those places. No one is there by choice. The anxiety is palpable. Anxious people talk—loudly and non-stop—to each other, on their phones, to anyone who will listen. Anxious people pace. They get angry. They cry; often in joy, but too often in grief. Hospital waiting lounges are a special purgatory.

Cath found an alcove with several comfy chairs down the hall and settled in. She had Sudoku. She had her Nook. She had her phone. She had four hours ahead of her.

She lasted several hours in her nook with her Nook. The grey and misty morning turned into a sunny September day. U-M Hospital has several buildings on campus, and in between the buildings is a large greenscape: trees, excellent shrubberies, the flowering plants of fall, picnic tables, and benches. Cath went outside. She still had her Sudoku, her phone, and her Nook. Comforting phone calls were made to her brother and sister-in-law, and to her parents, as well as mine.

Meanwhile, back in surgery, my team was involved in the dissection and resection of my face. You may recall that the final margins established formed a rough square about 2½ inches on each side. The surgeons decided to go a little larger than that. Take a regular 3 x 5 index card. Tear an inch off of the long end. Now, hold it up to your face with one edge right up against the front of your ear and another edge right at the top of your ear. That was the surgical field.

Skin, in that part of one's face, is between 1–2 mm thick. One square inch of skin contains about 50–60,000 melanocytes. Those, of course, are the rat-bastards that caused me to be in the hospital in the first place. One square inch of facial skin has about 650 sweat glands and perhaps 1,300 nerve endings. In addition, there are plenty of blood vessels in the area, 20 or more, which is why faces bleed so much when you nick yourself.

Underneath the seven layers of skin, there is plenty of other stuff as well. Muscles, fascia layers, tendons, bone—as Psalm 139 says, "Wonderfully and fearfully made."

Connective tissues, circulatory tissues, nervous tissues—Dr. Moyer and his team wanted to preserve as much of the underlayment as possible. Facial surgery is touchy stuff. You can't just peel off a layer of skin like a chicken thigh and call it good. The surgeons needed to most delicately remove the cancer-laden layers of skin, whilst keeping everything else as intact as possible. I have become accustomed to the nerves and muscles and blood vessels which make up the left side of my face. Lacking nerves and muscles and blood vessels, the side of my face would take on the appearance of one-too-many Hollywood facelifts. My plan was that when the surgery was complete, I would have a normal-looking, cancer-free face.

After three hours of waiting, Cath moved back into the waiting area. Still populated by nervous people, she wanted to be near the clerk-lady with the phone. Three and one-half hours after I was wheeled back, Cath received word that the team was finishing their work and that all had gone according to plan. A member of the surgical team would be out shortly to speak with her, she was told, and when I was awake, she'd be called back to the recovery area.

Melanoma: It Started With a Freckle

Another thirty minutes passed. A surgical resident came out to speak with her. He ushered her into one of several tiny rooms located along one wall of the waiting area. The room, Cath said, smelled of sweaty, scared people. It was so small and claustrophobic, Cath said, that you felt as if your personal space was invaded just by the surgeon walking into the phone-booth-sized cubicle.

"Your husband did great," said the surgical resident. "He tolerated the procedure well, no issues with anesthesia, we got out everything we needed to get out, and the closing—all the plastic surgery work—looks great. They sent tissue samples to the lab and they came back clean as can be. Your husband should have a very good plastic surgery result. He's starting to stir a bit in the recovery area so you'll be able to see him very soon."

Four hours and fifteen minutes to the moment after I had my pre-op meltdown, Cath was brought back into the recovery area. I was dressed in a pair of sweats I brought along. I sipped some Cran•Apple juice. That chilled little bottle of Ocean Spray juice through a straw was one of the finest beverages I've ever consumed. My face felt fine.

My right eye, on the other hand, was incredibly painful. It felt as if someone had dragged a shard of glass across my cornea in an effort to get me to answer "Is it safe?"

The recovery nurse asked how I felt. I told her about my eye. I mentioned the word "agony" and may have used the phrase "This hurts like a son of a bitch."

She said, "Yeah, that happens sometimes. Might have been the way your face was pressing on the table during surgery. Might have been a little piece of dried, crusty tear that couldn't get swept away by a blink before you were medicated. Want a Tylenol?"

"You feel ready to go? Here's your jacket. Let's get you in the wheel-chair. Okay, Mrs. Stanley? You know the way out? Okay, then. Bye"

I felt as if I was one step away from ripping my eyeball from my face and this nurse was hustling me out of post-op. In all the time I spent as a patient over my course of treatment, this was the first direct worker I came in contact with who seemed completely separated from the idea that patients are the reasons why a health care provider goes into healthcare. No call to the doctor about my eye. No eye drops. No ice pack. No "Where are you parked, Mrs. Stanley?"

Do you remember the scene in the old movie *Kiss of Death* when Richard Widmark's character Tommy Udo shoves the old lady in the wheelchair down a flight of stairs, cackling manically all the while? That was this nurse.

No matter. Cath knew the way. I sat in my wheelchair and Cath started to push my 170 pounds down a long series of halls. I felt as if I was in maze. The last third of the trip was uphill. Cath found the car. Cath helped me in. Cath got behind the wheel and we drove away.

She left the wheelchair in the parking lot.

In the car, I got a first glimpse of my face. As Cath described it, with the pressure bandage on my head, I looked like Alfalfa suffering from a very bad toothache. My teeth were fine. My eye had me scrunched over in pain. Tears on my face, eyeball throbbing, I dozed. Cath called my parents to let them know all was well and we were on our way home.

When I awoke on the northbound freeway, I decided I should call my parents and let them know that everything was fine. Cath handed me the phone. I dialed. I spoke with my Mom. I spoke with my Dad. I hung up. I dozed. I awoke. I decided to call my Dad and let him know everything went well. Indeed, thanks to modern pharmacology, no recollection existed that I had spoken with my Dad. Mom, yes. Dad? Not so much.

As we pulled into our driveway, a massive need to urinate overcame me. The car had barely stopped moving when I opened the door and clambered out. I trotted across the garage and pulled open the mud room door. I walked past the bathroom. I walked across the kitchen. Ignoring a left turn which would have taken me upstairs to another bathroom, I instead turned right and walked towards the doors leading to the deck. I opened the doors and walked out into my backyard.

I strode purposefully to a large sugar maple that sits in the center of our deck. I pulled down the front of my sweatpants. Looking down, I noted that upon my re-dressing at the hospital, I decided to go commando for the drive home. I proceeded to train Terence upon the tree. As I stood there urinating against a tree in our fenced-in backyard, I noticed that Cath was standing in the doorway.

"Watcha doin?" she asked. Her head was tilted at a quizzical angle.

"I had to pee."

"Uh, out here? You walked right past the bathroom."

"Um. Yeah. I don't know. I got nothing, babe. Seemed like a good idea at the time," I said.

"Maybe we should just sit out here on the deck for a while when you're done. It's a really nice day. Can I get you anything? A snack? Something to drink?"

It was a lovely late afternoon in fall. Cool, but not cold. Sunny, with plenty of fluffy stratocumulus clouds up in the lovely Michigan sky.

"Nah, I'm good. Thanks. Yeah, let's just sit," I said.

Settling into a deck chair, I looked at my reflection in the big glass windows which separate den from deck. In my fleece jacket, wearing a woolen ear flapper hat, I thought, "Hmm, more Elmer Fudd than Alfalfa."

"Love you, babe. Thanks for being with me through all this," I said.

"Well, I love you right back. And where else would I be?" said Cath.

I woke up on the deck several hours later. The sun was thinking about setting. Cath was inside getting dinner together. I remembered: how nice it was that I was home.

In the Arms of Hypnos

Sleep. That's what I did during my first post-operative days. After I peed against the tree in our backyard, Cath and I sat on our deck in the warmth of the early September sun. I dozed. I awoke, alone on the deck, wrapped in fleece and a now-ill-fitting Elmer Fudd earflap hat, as Cath napped in the house. Indeed, it had been a long day for her. Easy for me, all I had to do was lay there, unconscious, on the OR table. I didn't even have to breathe. Thanks to the paralyzing agent succinylcholine during anesthesia and the endotracheal tube attached to a ventilator, I didn't even have to breathe for myself.

I made a cup of tea and went back out on the deck. I watched, fully enthralled, as the dark red leaves of the Japanese maple fell to the ground. Nothing like a 5 am wake-up, a panic attack, 5 hours of surgery, and two point five hours of drive-time in the car to make one appreciate the miracle of the deciduous tree. I may have watched for minutes. It may have been many minutes. My eye was still exquisitely painful.

All I really recall was that I awoke again as the evening sun had dipped behind the house. Despite my arctic level get-up—fleece jacket, sweater, and Elmer Fudd hat—I was chilled. So was my mug of tea, barely touched, on the deck beside my chair.

Cath made soup for dinner. I ate a bit. Part of my brain was telling me I was starving but I was lacking in my normal zeal for a meal. The reality, as I raised my spoon to my mouth, was that the meds from surgery had so dried out my mucus membranes that I barely had enough saliva to fog a mirror. Food could wait.

By now, my eye was less painful. My face was pain-free. Hard to believe, but for all the surgery, the careful dissection of 25% of my face's surface, the removal of a considerable amount of underlying tissue, my face was essentially pain-free. I've had more discomfort from a simple burn in the kitchen.

I found it easy to follow the post-op instructions.

"Do not turn your head."

"No bending over."

"Ice. Apply as needed."

TV seemed the obvious choice. Propping my head up with a traveler's neck pillow, I settled in to watch TV. I awoke after several hours to Cath telling me it was time to go to bed.

Wandering upstairs, I contemplated my choice of pain medications. I needed to decide between regular items on the house menu: Darvocet or Motrin, or the chef's special—Vicodin. I hate the way that Vicodin makes everything flow in and out of focus. It's as if you've done tequila shots until you've gotten the spins, but with none of the fun or nausea. I broke a Vicodin in half. I figured if I didn't fall asleep within ten minutes, I would take the other half.

I had a reading pillow. I had codeine in my system. I had clean teeth. I had flannel pajama pants and a T-shirt. I had my nightstand lamp on. I had a book in my lap. When I awoke several hours later, needing to visit the loo, the lamp was still on, the book was still in my lap, and Cath was asleep beside me. As I stumbled to the bathroom, I caught a glimpse of myself in the mirror. With the pressure bandage around the side of my head, and another set of bandages across the top to hold the main bandage in place, I looked like Mr. Magoo with a severe toothache.

It was a sunny day on Tuesday morning when I woke. After cancer surgery, to awaken at home is the greatest of feelings. This was a lovely day. I did a quick inventory. Fingers and toes? They wiggled upon command. Neck and head? Sore, but not throbbing. After any bike race in which I crashed I've had much worse discomfort.

Vision? Aha. Turn torso (no twisting of the neck, remember) towards the window and the eyes don't want to focus when told. Turn torso back again? Yep, eyes are definitely not cooperating. Look far, then look close? Ah, no. Must be the drugs.

"Would you like any breakfast?" says Cath from the bathroom.

"Yes, please. Oatmeal."

"Got it. Don't forget, I'm going to work today so your Dad is coming by to hang out with you."

"Ah. No worries. My Dad is going to Davey-sit."

"Well, we all decided that someone should be with you today and tomorrow."

"We all? What mean 'we all'? I do not recall this discussion," I said.

"No, you wouldn't. You, my sweet man, were asleep on the couch."

"Oh, so you guys sorted this out on the phone last night?"

"No, sweetie. They stopped by to see you."

"Oh."

"And your oatmeal's ready. I'm leaving for work. Your Dad will be here around nine. You two stay out of trouble. See you after lunch. I'm doing a half-day. Love you."

After dressing in sweats and a hoodie, I looked at myself, a good look, in the mirror. I had an elastic band circling my skull around the top and bottom. I had another one, like a sweatband, around the circumference of my skull. I had a large pressure bandage on the left side of my face. It covered an area about five inches by five inches. The bandage was the size of a Big Boy double-decker hamburger. By seriously taxing my Vicodin-limited peripheral vision, I could see the edge of the bandage. I stopped peering around that corner. It made me dizzy.

I dabbed at the bandage. I pressed on it. No pain. I palpated the surgical site until I felt metal instead of tissue—the staples holding Dr. Moyer's work together. I felt forward, following the staple line, until I ran out of staples. The staples stopped just shy of my temple, at the hairline.

I worked my way back, until I got to the top of my ear. The staples took a 90-degree southward turn, straight down to the bottom of my ear lobe. There, they did a one-eighty and began their climb up and behind my ear. The staple stopped on the lump of my temporal bone-the spot where one's glasses rest. I went to the garage and grabbed a steel tape measure. I had 5¾ inches of suture line which the staples in my face were holding together. My incision was indeed a mirror image square root sign, with my ear in the little $\sqrt{}$ vee.

I felt the fronts of both shoulders. Dr. Moyer had said that if he needed a skin graft, he'd pull the tissue from my shoulder. If a graft had been discussed during the recovery room conference, it had not been stored in my data banks. Nope, nothing. My facial skin still had enough elasticity to stretch over a hole on my skull big enough through which to pass one's fist.

I was seated at the kitchen table and eating my oatmeal when Dad knocked on the garage door and walked in. I was nursing my day's only cup of coffee. Caffeine raises blood pressure and speeds heart rates. Bad for bloodless, bruise-less, painless healing. So far, being both bruise and pain-free, I planned on leading the league in patient compliancy. Mort had the Sunday *New York Times* in his hand.

"Hey, I brought you some reading material. That is, if you can stay awake. You were pretty zonked when we stopped by yesterday. You did know that? That we came by?"

"Um, I was not aware. But I was informed after the fact. This morning."

"Yeah, you don't blow off four hours of anesthesia any too fast. After my bypass, I couldn't keep track of time for a couple days post-op. Didn't really know what day it was. How's your face? Hurt? Throbbing? Nothing? Some combination thereof?"

"Truth be told, I feel fine. Nothing. I've felt worse after bike crashes. Way worse after I broke my collarbone."

"That's good surgical technique, then. That's why you were in there for so long. Let's watch Regis and Kelly. You take the couch so you can just lean back and go to sleep. I'll take the easy chair. Remember, you need to sleep sitting up."

An interesting tone accompanied these instructions. Part caring and concerned dad, part doctor with fifty years of medical/surgical experience under his belt. Forty years past that adolescent time of my life when I challenged everything my father said, I was now very happy and willing to have someone else in charge of my life for a few hours.

When I awoke, several hours later, there was no more Regis, the sound was off, and my Dad was dozing in the comfy chair. I looked at my watch. It was past noon. I'd been asleep for several hours.

I warmed up the beef and barley soup Cath had made the previous night for dinner which I had not eaten. My father and I ate soup. My father took his *Times* and went home. I was instructed to not do anything stupid until my wife got home.

"And don't do anything stupid once she gets home, either," said Dad as he left shortly before one.

My post-op, thankfully, was less than thrilling.

It was a sunny, cool day. I had a book. My mother had heard of my sore eye. She thoughtfully checked out a large print version of *Heat* for my post-op reading. The author, Bill Buford, a *New Yorker* writer, indentured himself to star chef Mario Batali for a series of articles on the restaurant business. He fell in love with the business, and moved to Italy to learn the secrets of Euro-style butchery.

Yes, a man who had undergone five hours of biopsy and five hours of major surgery was sitting on his deck, wrapped in fleece and wearing an Elmer Fudd hat, whilst reading a book on how to become an old-fashioned butcher.

Irony noted.

I am not sure when Cath arrived home. I awoke on the deck, upright, and with my head held firmly vertical by my neck pillow. My book was across my chest, and the sun was starting to sink behind the roofline of our house. It was chilly. I was hungry.

I walked into the house. Cath was asleep on the couch with her feet poking out from under the afghan. I wriggled her be-socked foot.

"Hey," I said. "You're home. How are you?"

"Huh? Wha? Oh, hey, you're awake," Cath said. "I saw you asleep out there. You looked so cozy, all snuggled down in all that fleece. Nice hat. Good choice with those earflaps. You didn't get cold out there, did you?"

"Nah. I was fine. I was reading and I just thought I'd rest for a second and, well, here we are. I'm still tired."

"Tired? Why should you be tired?" said Cath as she patted the couch, an invitation to join her.

"All you've done is sleep."

She laughed.

"I was the one up all last night, watching you sleep. I'm the one that's tired. I love you, you know."

"I love you back. And thank you. I can't imagine doing this alone."

"I'm your wife. I love you. Where else would I be?"

I leaned forward to hug my wife, my Cath. She pushed me back up-right.

"No bending over. No twisting your head. No exertion. Remember?" she said.

"Ah, crap," I said. "So much for the second half of my post-op rehab plan."

You, Sir, Are So Good-lookin'

Truly, what I did for the rest of the first post-op week was sleep, and then sleep some more. It was a beautiful September and I spent more time wrapped in the arms of Hypnos than I did wrapped in the arms of my wife. So simple. Make tea. Bundle up in fleece because even temps in the low 60s felt chilly. Sit in a deck chair with my neck pillow. Read my large print version of *Heat* for a few moments. Sleep. Awaken. Repeat. Dr. Moyer's injunction about "no exercise" was not needed. I didn't want to do anything. I was deeply fatigued. I am not unfamiliar with extreme fatigue.

In my twenties, I was a full-time bicycle racer. We traveled from town to town, my three buddies and I, in my 4WD Toyota Tercel wagon and a VW Jetta. A typical race might be 50 miles long; 50 laps around a one mile city circuit with four to eight corners. The race would start out at a demonic pace, perhaps 32 mph for the first five miles, and then settle into a more reasonable 28–30 mph for the next 40 miles. The problem was that at every corner, just like in an F1 auto race, we hit the brakes down to 23 mph, and as we exited the turn, we had to sprint back up to speed. That's a lot of sprints. As for the last 5–10 miles, the speed ratcheted back up to 32–35 mph.

You ride a bicycle at that tempo for a few hours, and by race's end, you're barely able to change clothes and pack up the car. Sometimes, you're too exhausted to eat, and it's work to shove down enough calories to make up for what was burned off in the race. Worse, when you arrive at the Motel 6 or Days Inn, you're completely spent, but your metabolism is still so ramped up, you're unable to fall asleep. Extreme fatigue is no stranger to my system. However, this drug-induced fatigue took "drained" to a new place.

Normally, I dream lucidly, vividly, and actively. I can feel myself fall asleep. There is a lot of swooping and gravity-defying in my dreams. In my dreams, I fly, I soar, I ski. My dreams are usually fun, usually colorful, and I usually remember them. Not now. My sleep mechanism was now like a giant electrical switch in *Young Frankenstein*. When Igor threw the switch, without warning, out go the lights. I slept without consciousness for hours, and I would awaken with no awareness of the passing of time.

On Thursday morning, the third post-op day, Cath donned her nurse's cap and removed the pressure bandage. She snuck a peek.

"This looks great," she said.

The fatigue was lifting. I walked about the backyard, admiring the trees and fallen leaves. I took the trash out to the curb and did not have to stop to catch my breath along the way. The dog accompanied me for brief walks to the street corner and back, a total distance of 200 yards. I could carry on a conversation about the high school tennis season with Aaron without stopping to "rest my eyes" in mid-sentence. I could now walk up the stairs without a rest stop on the landing. When not in motion, however, I still fell asleep, deeply asleep, without warning. Note I said "lifting", not "lifted."

My surgery was on a Monday. Eight days later, I was scheduled for inspection. My father and I drove the 65 minutes from Flint to Dr. Moyer's luxurious office in Livonia. Still such an odd feeling, that office. It was as if one had stepped into a Tiffany's advertisement. There were people waiting to be seen who had been through life-threatening conditions and for whom surgery was well and truly life-saving. Seated right next to them were already lovely women for whom facial surgery seemed to be a hobby.

I was seen promptly.

Dr. Moyer walked into the room and said, "Heard you had a little pre-op freak-out? Nerves caught up with you?"

I relayed the story of the traffic, and the lady at check-in, and the gum.

He nodded.

"Makes sense to me. You're not the first. I'm kind of like you, I like to be in charge and I like to know what's what. No surprise. I don't know that I'd be any better. It's cancer. It's scary. This wasn't a nose job, you know?

"Let's see how I did, okay?"

He carefully removed the bandages. I watched him in the reflection from the exam room window. He stepped back. He tilted his head; first this way, then that. He furrowed his brows and leaned forward. He truly did look like an artist analyzing his painting. If he would have held up his thumb, I would not have been surprised.

I could feel his breath. He felt along the suture line. He palpated behind my ear, under my jawline, along my hairline. He stepped back and put his hands in his lab coat pocket and spoke.

"This is terrific. You did great in OR. That made my job easy. And I'll tell you, you heal fast. This looks super. We can take the staples out today, for sure. My PA," he nodded at the woman beside him, "will pull those staples out and I'll be right back. Need to go inject a bit of Botox. Cancer. Wrinkles. That's my practice."

We laughed. He left. The PA pulled a staple removal kit from a cabinet.

"You don't want these staples, do you?" she asked a touch of yuck in her voice.

"Um, no. Gunked-up surgical staples? I'll pass. Why? Do some people keep their staples?"

She arched her eyebrows, rolled her eyes and said, "Oh, you'd be real surprised at some of the things Dr. Moyer's patients have asked me to save for them."

"My Dad's a retired proctologist, so...," I said.

"He ever get asked to save the ... ? Never mind, moving on" she said. "Okay, sit up straight, hold still for a few minutes and we're done."

I could hear the faint click of her tweezers closing around a staple. I felt the slightest tug. I heard a quiet "ting" as she dropped the staple in a plastic tray. And we were done.

"This is healing really nicely. In a few months, you won't even see the scar," she said. "Well, you will behind the ear, because that's where everything is anchored, but even that scar won't be big. Doctor used some facelift techniques on you. Yep, this looks really good."

"How many..."

"Stitches?" she finished for me. "You guys. Men always want to know. You all keep track. Looks like he used about 20, maybe 25 staples, to close it up. How many have you had?"

"Counting these, I'm right around 200 stitches and staples. And everyone's a story, lemme tell you."

"I'm good. Really."

She held up her hand.

"No stories. I'll get Dr. Moyer."

As he walked into the room, Moyer stopped in doorway, looked at me sitting sideways in the exam chair, and whistled.

"You, sir, are sooooooooooo good lookin'," he said.

"Seriously, though, impressive. Your site came together quickly. You're fast. No swelling. No bruising. Not even a hint of discoloration. And that suture line is matched up perfectly. That's what happens when you keep your head upright. When you don't twist your neck. Good stuff.

"Okay, here's the deal. I'll see you once more, next week. Stop at the desk on the way out. They'll give you orders for an MRI. We'll get that scheduled for you today before you leave. How's your pain? Do you need any more meds?"

"Meds? No, I'm good. I've only used like two of the Vicodin. I tell you, you were right, road rash hurts way worse. Uh, MRI? No one's mentioned an MRI before."

I was confused and a little nervous.

"The MRI? Yeah, we always order an MRI for facial melanoma. Need to make sure that nothing's metastasized. Standard. And before you get all frantic on me, in your case, I'd say there is about a 99.9% chance that you have none."

"I guess that makes sense, but geez, an MRI? Is that really necessary?" I asked.

"Yes. Yes, it is. We need to make sure. All this work and time, we need to be absolutely certain. MRIs don't hurt. They're non-invasive. You've got a machine right in your hometown. So what's the big deal?"

"I don't know. I mean, that tube, and kind of being locked in and all that…"

"Ah, some latent claustrophobia. Okay, I get that. You are claustrophobic, right? You're in the machine about 20 minutes for this. It's noisy, even with headphones on, and it's cramped. We can't have you moving around. So, if you think you'll have issues, I'll write for some Ativan. It works great, but it'll make you woozy. You'll need a driver for the ride home."

I thought back to my love-hate relationship with the cramped tubes of air travel.

"Yes.

"Write the Ativan."

Panic Travels at 134 MPH

My father joined me, two days later, for Wednesday morning's drive to the MRI lab. He walked into the house and I was staring at two pill bottles. One bottle had a few Xanax in it; a remnant of my last plane trip. I do not like to not be in charge. I don't like enclosed spaces. Planes fail on both accounts.

In the other bottle, 4 Ativan rattled around. I felt like Hamlet, staring at a skull. *To Xanax, or Ativan, that is the question? Whether shouldst thou take the Xanax and just be chill, or down the Ativan and be thus woozy the remains of the day?*

I hate being woozy. I spent enough time being woozy in the past week. I opted for a Xanax.

Dad drove the ten minutes to the lab. I filled out the paperwork and was promptly ushered into the lab. It was cold. I sat on the edge of the MRI table. This was touted as an "open" MRI.

With a standard MRI machine, you lay on a table and the tech rolls you into a steel tube which resembles a small missile silo. A small blanket or hand towel is placed over your eyes. Since the machine's wall is fractions of an inch away from your nose, the sensation of hiding under the covers is not inappropriate. Even for those not claustrophobic, it is highly taxing to the nervous system. In other words, most people are about ready to scream "Get Me the Hell Out of Here" before the exam has even begun.

The open machine more closely resembles a partially closed panini press. It is open on either side of your head to the exam room. Some fresh air does move through the space. However, the machine is still millimeters away from your face and you cannot turn your head. To the claustrophobic, the issue of open vs. closed is akin to root canal or wisdom tooth removal.

The tech was a very calm man, also named Dave. Every day, he dealt with people in a near-panic state. In a gentle voice, he asked, "I see you're a bit claustrophobic. Did you take the Ativan?"

"No, sir. I opted for some Xanax, instead. I hate that woozy, dizzy Ativan haze."

"Ah, okay. Sure. Got it. Let's talk for a moment. The procedure will take about 20 minutes or so. MRIs are completely painless and harmless. We don't use x-rays. We use magnetism to create the images the doctors need. I know that these procedures are nerve-wracking. You're already not feeling all that well, or the doctors suspect something's not quite right, and when we slide you into the tube…So this is tough.

"I know 'cause I had one. Promise, I won't do anything without telling you first. We want you to be as comfortable as can be, okay? We have headphones, you can listen to music, we'll talk with each other. It'll be okay. My patients usually like to chat at first, and as the procedure goes on, it's not uncommon for them to doze off. It is a bit noisy in there, but it's a consistent noise, like being in a window seat on a plane.

"Oh, and there is also a button for you so you're in charge. If things get really uncomfortable in there, and I've had an MRI, remember, so I get you, you hit that button, see, right there, like a *Jeopardy* buzzer, and I'll drop what I'm doing and we can talk it through. Okay? Sounds good? Let's do this. Swing your feet up, lay your head down on this neck massager and we'll roll you in."

I lay back, not without some trepidation. Twenty minutes isn't long, I thought. 1200 seconds. About 400 breaths, I thought, as I lay there on the table. I can do this. I have to do this.

"Now, here, put on the headphones. You hear the music? Good, just listen to the music. I'm going to cover your eyes with this clean towel. It's just easier this way. No one knows why. You'll be more comfortable if you happen to open your eyes and all you see is towel. Trust me on this, Dave.

"Okay, you're comfy? Well, reasonably comfy? Close your eyes, listen to some tunes, take a few deep breaths, it'll be a few moments 'til we can talk. After I roll you in, I need to get up to the control room. And in.. we.. go…"

No five year old on the first day of kindergarten has every held onto a parent's hand as tightly as I squeezed that panic button. I stretched my neck, knowing I wouldn't be able to move my head for the next twenty minutes. I can do this, I thought. Xanax don't fail me now.

"Hey! How ya doing?"

I heard Dave's friendly voice through the headphones.

"Um, you know, well. I've been better but this is not too bad…"

A wave of panic flew at 60 meters per second from my toes to my nose. Indeed, nerve impulses do travel at 30 miles per hour. At that moment, I was fully capable of a 200 kilograms clean and jerk. A nine second 100 meter dash. Xanax or not, I was revved.

"You need to get me out of here!"

"Okay, Dave. Talk to me. What's going on?"

"I can't stay in here. I don't know where the Hell it came from. I felt okay, and all of sudden, I'm ready to rip this machine apart to get outta here. I'm trying to take some deep breaths but all I get is panic. I'm sorry, Dave, but there's no fucking way, I mean..."

"Okay, hang on. Don't wreck my machine, bro. I'm coming down."

I heard a door, some squeaks of his shoes on the floor, and then he grabbed my hand.

"I'm right here. Now, talk to me."

I tried to breathe slowly enough to get words out. It occurred to me, after the fact, that he was taking my pulse, racing, and feeling my palms, cold and sweaty.

"I'm gonna roll you out, we'll talk for a minute and calm down. Maybe we'll try again."

The machine hummed and whirred, the table retracted, and I felt the fluorescent lights on my face through the towel. I removed the towel as I sat up.

"I'm sorry, Dave. I don't know what happened."

"Well, um, you panicked, that's what happened. Happens enough. Hey, I thought you took some Xanax?"

"I took one."

"Not enough. I mean, I'm not a doctor, but that's why they always write Ativan. Xanax just isn't strong enough. You got anymore Xanax with you? No, huh? Did you fill the script for Ativan? Good.

"Alright, here's what we'll do. 'Cause there is no way, as wound up as you are, that you'll be able to go back in there. We'll just be causing you more headache and the rest of the patients will be running way late. Lemme check the schedule for tomorrow.

"I know we have a few openings. I'll find you the opening, if you'll take Ativan. Deal? We'll do this thing tomorrow. It's gotta get done. You can do this. Just take the drugs. Okay? Just take the drugs. Here's your appointment time.

"Dude. Just take the drugs."

"I'll take the drugs. Sorry about all this, Dave. I'll take the drugs. Promise."

With a great deal of chagrin, I headed into the lobby. Dad was reading in the chair.

"That was fast."

"Yeah, well, about that. We need to come back tomorrow. I sort of freaked out in the machine. The Xanax wasn't enough."

Dad looked at me over the tops of his glasses.

"No, it's not. That's why Moyer wrote the Ativan."

"Well, why didn't you say something? You're a doctor."

"True, I am a doctor, but… one, you didn't ask me and two, I am not your doctor. So what's the plan?"

"Well, Dad, the tech got me a slot for tomorrow at ten. I had to promise to take the Ativan. I feel like I could use the Ativan right now. So, are you free to drive in the morning?"

Singing in the MRI

Just before 10 am the next morning, Mort drove his drug addled and slightly woozy 48-year-old son back to the lab. I approached the woman at the desk like a student who had been sent to the principal.

"I'm really sorry about yesterday. I know that screws up the schedule..."

"Ah, don't worry about it," she said. "That happens all the time. ALL the time. Well, at least once or twice a week. We sort of plan on it."

She looked at me with the look of a teenager asking someone to buy her some beer and whispered, "You did take the Ativan this time?"

I felt my face redden.

"Oooooh yeeeeaaah. I took the Ativan."

Dave, the technician, held the door for me. As we walked back, he gently put his hand on my back.

"You did take the Ativan, didn't you?"

I blushed again.

"Yeah. I took the Ativan. Sorry about all that yesterday. The surgery. The MRI. Some semi-latent claustrophobia. Who knew?"

We walked into the room. I looked around. It looked like a mini-version of the control room from the movie *WarGames*. I sat on the MRI table again.

Dave explained the procedure.

"Right. You're more relaxed. I can see it. You're gonna do great today. Okay. I'll have you lie down and put on the headphones. Were you good with that station? I'll give you the button, cover your eyes with a towel, and I'll roll you in. Now, we never got this far yesterday, but there's two parts to the exam. The first part takes most of the exam. That's the general views. The second part takes about three minutes and it involves the injection of some contrast medium. So, I can start the line now, and then pop down and inject the dye, won't even have to roll you out, or I can roll you out, shoot the dye, and then roll you in. Your choice."

I sat up a little straighter.

"Contrast medium? IV? Hold on a sec. Nobody said anything about an IV."

"Deep breaths, there, Dave. C'mon, don't freak out on me now. No big deal. Remember, I had one of these a while back for a bad headache. I've done hundreds for patients. Doesn't hurt. You have a shellfish allergy? No? Good.

"You won't hardly feel the dye going in. You're not gonna wet yourself, or anything like that. Some patients say their groin gets warm, but not everybody. You might. It's the dye. But I promise, you're not peeing your pants.

"Dave, this is the easy part. It's like the two minute warning. I shoot the dye, and you're almost done. And they really need those contrast shots. I mean, geez, look at your veins. They're huge. You should see some of the little old ladies I have to do."

"Ah, yeah, no," I said. "I mean, I'm fine with IVs and stuff. I've had plenty. You caught me by surprise is all. Didn't know anyone would be shooting contrast in. Gimme a second. I'll be fine. Let's do the IV now."

I leaned back onto the table. It was chilly. I slid on the headphones. Some random pop music was playing. The button was placed in my right hand. I closed my eyes. The light seemed to dim as Dave placed a towel over my eyes. I tried to breathe deep down into my legs and back out my nose. A few breaths and I felt Dave take my left wrist.

"Putting in the IV. This'll be easy. These are great veins. You'll feel a little prick in 3, 2, 1. There. Done."

I felt the familiar pressure of a large bore needle sliding into the back of my hand. I heard the tear of paper as he ripped several pieces of tape to secure the IV in place.

I heard a distant Dave say, "In you go. Be right with you. Gotta get to my work station."

I heard a faint whrrr and the table rolled smoothly into the tube. I concentrated on feeling the cool air from the open sides waft onto my ears. It was tolerable. I thought back.

"This is definitely better than the last biopsy. And definitely better than more surgery."

"And we're back," I heard Dave say in the headphones.

"Here's the drill. It gets noisy. The actual workings of the machine rotate around your head. Every time you hear a set of clunks, that's more rotation. The clicking sounds, that's the actual image. And no, I don't remember how many clicks and clunks until you're done. When I had mine done, the Ativan knocked me on my ass, and I, uh, sorta fell asleep. You're okay, aren't you? Don't move… And we're rolling."

I lay there in the tube, feeling the cool air on the sides of my head, listening to a million dollar piece of precision instrumentation clunk and chunk around my head as if it were a poorly tuned motorcycle.

I thought, "Hmm, I should be panic-stricken right now. But I'm not. Oh. Right. Two milligrams of Ativan."

In my head, I started singing along with a song on the headphones. I heard a voice.

"Uh, Dave? Dave! No singing in the machine. It moves your jaw and that screws up the imaging. Seriously. You were singing in there."

"Oops. Sorry. I'll stop."

"We need to back up for that last shot, then you'll have about two more minutes' worth. Then I'll come down, shoot you up, another couple minutes of imaging, and we're done."

A moment later, I felt Dave's hand grasp my left wrist. "Here's the contrast medium. Some people feel this medium a little chilly as it goes in. Some feel it warm. You'll probably get a metallic taste in your mouth, like touching your tongue to a battery. That goes away pretty fast. You're doing great this time. Nice comeback. I gotta run. Hang in."

It was a spot-on description. A bit of chill in my hand and arm, the taste of a nine volt battery on my tongue, and then Dave in my ear.

"Hey, you're a teacher, huh? Whaddaya teach? You can talk. I still need a moment."

"Science, Dave. Bio, anatomy, zoology, some chem, and the odd physics class when needed."

"How about I burn you a CD of your images? Take it back to class; show your kids you really have a brain in there? Okay, no talking. Hold still. A couple more clicks. And we're done. YES! Great job, boss! Great job. Thanks for toughing this out. Be right there. Don't move until I tell you. Last guy who sat up too fast needed a couple stitches to close up his forehead."

A whrrr and a grumble, the lights brightened, and I heard Dave say, "And we're clear! Gimme your hand and I'll pull the cath out. Nice."

I hopped off the table. I stuck out my right hand.

"Thanks for putting up with me, Dave. Really appreciate it."

He grabbed my hand, reached out with his other arm. I pulled him in. Bro-hug.

"Glad to help, man. Glad to help," he said. "Lemme grab that CD for you before we forget. You see your doctor when? Monday? He'll have the report by then. Hope everything keeps working out for you. And really, yours wasn't the worst freak-out. Sorry. Not even close."

I walked out of the exam area with my CD in hand. Dad was awake and flipping through a golf magazine.

125

"Go better this time?" he asked.

"Yep, saved by modern pharmacology. And the tech burned me CD of the images. We can check it out at home."

Mort said, "Is this my cue, I start singing 'If I Only Had a Brain'…?"

"Hehe. Very funny. You're driving. I still feel like I just knocked back a few shots of Jack Daniels. I'm hungry. How long was I back there?"

Dad looked at his watch. "A little over an hour, I guess. Seem longer? Or shorter?"

"Shorter, I guess. I might have dozed off. Not sure. He did have to stop for a few minutes, though."

"Hmm, why's that?" asked Dad.

"I, er, started singing along with a song on the headphones."

"You're kidding," said Dad.

"I kid you not. I thought I was singing along in my head. Or maybe humming," I said. "But no, Dave said I was, uh, singing."

"Beats the screaming I heard you doing yesterday. Where we going for lunch? And yes, I'm driving."

Part Five
The Encore, and
Meet and Greet in the Lobby

You Should be Tired

My MRI was completed on a Thursday. On Friday morning, eleven days post-operatively, our landline rang.

"Hi, this is Dr. Moyer's office. I'm Dr. Moyer's PA, the one who took out your staples and stitches? Yes. I have your MRI results. He says to tell you that your report looks great. When we saw you for the staple removal last week, we all agreed that things were healing faster than expected.

"Since then, have you had any drainage? Has the site separated anywhere? No? That's great. Any pain; anything at all to report? No?"

"I feel great. Pretty normal. Nothing hurts. Nothing oozes. Very cool, all things considered."

"Now, ordinarily," she went on, "we'd like to see you one more time, but since you have a doctor in the family and your wife is a nurse and we're in close contact with Dr. Barkey, unless you have a compelling reason to drive down from Flint to our office, Dr. Moyer and I agree that there's no real need for you to make the trip. You good with that?"

"Good with that? I'm frickin' great with that."

"Nice. Okay, then. You, sir, are just two weeks post-op. Here's the deal. One, we don't want you back in the weight room for one month. Even though everything is well-sealed, you go deep on a squat, really clench down on your traps and delts, you could tear Dr. Moyer's work open. Then we're back to scar revisions. We hate scar revisions. So just don't. No weights for another thirty days. No, don't start. This is not a discussion. Got it?"

"Yes, ma'am. No weights for another thirty days. Roger that."

"Two, you can ride your bike, but again, no big efforts for one month. Same deal. And for all that is holy in this world, be careful. Do not crash. If you crash, that's just making extra work for everyone. You have an indoor trainer? Maybe just ride indoors, okay? Get it? Good."

"Yes, ma'am. Cautious Dave, that's me."

"Three, you can go back to work on Monday. Take it easy. I get the sense that you're not one of those teachers that just sits behind the desk. Well, for the next few weeks, you might want to be one of those teachers.

"Mr. Stanley, how are you feeling, in general?"

"I'm tired. I'm a lot better than I was those first few days, but I still crash like some old geezer," I said. "I go to bed early, wake up late, nap more than I have in maybe ever. I'm way better, but still…"

"You're tired? Yeah, that'll happen. Surgery is hard work. There's a lot of insult to the body. What with the anesthesia, we invade your body, major healing process, yep, you should be tired. You might want to plan a nap into your afternoon. You had a long surgery, with lots of work done; ten, twelve days ago. Might want to think about, when you come home from school, grabbing a nap for a while before anything else. That's what a lot of our facelift patients do, and you had lots more done than a facelift."

"My wife and both noticed," I put in, "my face definitely looks, um, snugger, on the left side, since the surgery. There's no swelling. We both see that some wrinkles are gone."

"Uh, yeah, sorry, but that'll go away. Hard to tell when, but since Dr. Moyer didn't anchor any of the skin back down along the way, like he would with a real facelift, that's just a temporary bonus. Enjoy.

"So, if anything happens, any questions, whatever, you have our post-op phone number, please call. But otherwise, be well. Here's where we set you free."

"Set me free?"

"Right, Dr. Barkey's in charge from here on out. The usual protocol is he'll see you twice this month, and then once a month for the next six months. He'll be looking at your operative site, for sure, but he'll also be doing a head to toe inspection. Melanoma really is that sneaky. After the first six months, he'll see you every other month for the rest of the year. After that, it's kind of up to him but my guess is, every other month for another 6 months. Then, he'll probably switch to once a quarter. Sound good? Good. Do yourself a favor, seriously, take it easy for the next few weeks at work."

My vacation was over. I was going back to work.

Back to Work;
My Bravest Student

Sunday night, I made sure my lunch was packed. I made an omelet for breakfast, which needed only to be microwaved at 6:00 am. My clothes were laid out. I'll go out on a limb here and say I chose khakis and a polo shirt. In bed by 9:00, I do recall that I fell asleep quite promptly. At this point in my recovery, two weeks in, I could still fall asleep like a man with a serious melatonin imbalance.

Monday morning, my feet hit the floor at 5:30 am. No snooze button this morning. Coffee-ed, showered, dressed, and breakfasted by 6:40, Cath hugged me, hugged me hard, as I headed towards the car.

"Have a great first day back, okay? I know you've been wanting this for a week. Enjoy this first day. Promise?"

"I promise," I said, as I hugged her back.

Feeling like a kid on the first day of school after summer vacation, I settled into the driver's seat, buckled my seatbelt and contemplated my radio presets. No sports talk radio, no NPR, no morning drive time rock for this commute. I put Christopher Parkening's Bach Prelude no. 1 in C major into the CD player. Classical guitar encourages introspection and Bach even more so. I had plenty of thoughts to keep me company.

I was anxious to see how things went with my guest teacher in charge for two weeks' time. I do like teaching. My students are great fun. I enjoy being around my colleagues. In my briefcase was a flash-drive containing my lesson plans for the coming week and the DVD from my MRI. My first day back, my lesson was "all about me"—me and melanoma.

I parked in the teacher's lot. I met up with several colleagues as I walked in. Lots of hugs, lots of good-ta-see-yas, lots of nice-to-have-you-backs. I got hugs from all of our front office staff and made my way to my classroom for the first time in two weeks.

Even at 7:15 am, with school not scheduled to start until 7:50 am, our halls had begun to fill with students. I may have set a faculty record for student high-fives as I walked down the hall, up the stairs, and further down another hall to my room. I reached my classroom and several students were sitting in our carpeted hall outside my door. They had Pop-Tarts and granola bars and some fruit. A few drank hot chocolate on this chilly late September morning.

"Oh My God, we are so glad you're back. That guy!"

"We heard you picked him. He was such a tool. He wouldn't let us talk in class; we had to ask permission to go to the bathroom a certain way. He was mean."

I thought to myself, "Perfect. A mean sub. Every teacher loves a mean sub."

I said to the kids, "We'll talk about all that once we get started this morning. I need to make some coffee and get my stuff together before the bell rings, okay?"

I wandered into my back room. Science teachers, we have a lot of "science-y stuff" to store so my classroom connects with the physics teacher's room next door via a shared storage room about the size of semi-trailer. I made some coffee and flipped through the files of student work that my guest teacher had collated for me. Standing back there, I heard students whispering, and not-so-much whispering.

"Stanley's back."

"Stan-Man's here?"

"Well, crap. He's back? Now we're gonna have to do, you know, real work."

The bell rang. I heard the rasping and clanging of chairs as students found their seats. I stood in the doorway at the back of the room with my coffee mug in hand. As I peeked around the storage room corner, with my remote control I turned on the SmartBoard, a computerized, interactive whiteboard/movie screen, at the front of the room. I stood silently and watched kids read the day's assignment on the PowerPoint screen at the front of the class.

It read:

TALK ABOUT STANLEY'S CANCER.

There was a momentary lull as the kids read the screen. I took advantage to walk to the front of the class. I hopped onto my demonstration table.

"Hey, how are you guys? You might not believe this, but it's good to be not dead, and it's good to be back here. Really. Even here is better than, well, you know, not, erm, being anywhere. You know, dead.

"I heard that Mr. Snape was pretty tough."

A moderately loud hub-bub began to arise. I held up my hand to slow down the onslaught.

Melanoma: It Started With a Freckle

"I know, I know. He's an old school kind of teacher. That's why I asked for him. Yes, I asked for him. See, you guys and me, we have a relationship. You all know what to expect from me, I have a pretty good idea of what I'm getting with you, we know we're gonna have to get along together all semester, so we understand that we're all in this together.

"But you guys and Mr. Snape, well, you both knew that in two weeks' time, he'd be moving on. So, he needed to be tough to keep you guys focused. He was doing exactly as I requested. We're still on schedule with our lessons, I was looking at your quizzes, they looked solid, so I'd say, you guys, whether you realized it or not, did great stuff together. Thank you.

"But, we can talk more about that stuff later, if you want. For the rest of today, I want to talk about me. Well, I want to talk about you guys, too. I want to talk about my cancer a little. I have a few slides to show you. I'm gonna ask you guys to nag your parents a little, and I want to talk about you guys and cancer, too."

In my classroom, I have a document camera. If you recall the opaque projectors of the old days, you have the idea. It has a digital camera which can focus on any object on the platen. The image travels to my computer, gets sent to a ceiling mounted projector, and then the image is seen on the large SmartBoard in the front of my classroom.

"Who wants to see my scar?" I asked.

"Me!"

"Yes!"

"Cool!"

"Argh, not in first hour!"

"Gross!"

The chorus traveled like the wave around the room. I walked to my work station, spun the camera around onto the left side of my face, and focused the camera on an up-close and personal image of my ear and the immediate area.

I craned my neck a teeny bit and I was able to see what my students saw. It was an extreme close-up of my face; a graying middle-aged man's face. The four foot tall image was slightly hairy and a bit splotchy. Through the center of the image ran, in the rough shape of a mirror-imaged square root sign, a purplish-red healing scar. I interposed pencil, eraser end foremost, between my face and the camera.

"My cancer, on the skin, anyways, was not quite this big."

I tapped the area in front of my tragus for emphasis. I tore an inch off of the long end of a three by five inch index card and held in over the operative site.

"This," I said, "was how much flesh and skin, right down to the bone, the doctors had to remove to give me a good chance that my skin cancer, my melanoma won't return. I lived in Texas. I spent twenty hours a week on a bike. I was outdoors all the time playing soccer and tennis. I never used sunscreen. Truth is, back then, no one wore sunscreen. This is what happens."

I traced my scar with the pencil eraser. I let the silence hang over the room.

"Okay, I want to show you guys something that I want you to nag your parents about. Go ahead, rat me out. I'm gonna show you guys some slides about the warning signs of skin cancer and melanoma. If you see anything like this on your moms and dads, uncles, aunts, whatever, you nag them to get it looked at by your doctor.

"Chances are, it'll be nothing, but 2% of the time, it'll be something. 2% sounds like nothing, doesn't it? But how many of you guys have parents that buy a MegaMillions ticket? Right, well, the odds of winning the MegaMillions is about 1 in 2 billion with a 'B', but you still buy that one dollar ticket? And the odds of white folks getting melanoma, that's about 1 in 50. So blame me, if you want, but nag 'em."

I ran through my slide show.

"Here, kids, are what you're looking for on Mom and Dad. The warning signs:"

A is for Asymmetry. If you draw a line through the growth, the halves are not mirror images.

B is for Border. The edges are erose or scalloped.

C is for Color. A growth with a variety of colors is bad.

D is for Diameter. Most melanomas are bigger than 0.25 inches.

E is for Evolving. Growing larger or out from the skin, changing color; any change needs to be investigated.

Along the way, yes, I included several slides, shown without warning, of the grotesque damage that melanoma can cause. I also included a brief film clip of noted melanoma victim Bob Marley, complete with a great version of *Lively Up Yourself*.

"Okay, now that we've seen the damage melanoma can do, and you're going home convinced that every little dot on your body, and every person you care about, is cancer and it's gonna gnaw off your face, piece by piece, lemme tell you a story."

I told them about my MRI freak-out. Hilarity ensues, at my expense, and the proper atmosphere is restored. I show them a few views of my brain. More hilarity ensues. My father would be proud of my students' ability to poke fun at their teacher.

I prop myself back on my demo table at the front of the room.

"I'm gonna ask you guys some questions about cancer and I want to ask you guys for a show of hands. You don't have to play if you don't want to. I don't have prizes for winners. I don't even have any parting gifts. I just want to ask you a few questions.

"Okay? Good. Now, remember, you don't have to play.

"This may be tough, but has anyone in here had cancer?"

A boy in the back raises his hand.

"Yeah. Me."

"Can you talk about it, Cody? You don't have to, you know."

"No, it's cool. I had kidney cancer when I was little. I was four, I think. I just remember always being in the hospital that year. It's really rare, they told me, but I got it. They ended up taking out my kidney. You know that scar on my back, Jake?"

Jake nods.

"You said you got that falling off a ladder or something when I asked you about it."

"Yeah, I lied. I don't like thinking about having cancer too much, so when you asked, I just lied. Sorry, dude."

"Oh, that's cool," said Jake. "Not about the cancer. I mean, cancer sucks, I mean, lying and everything. Whatever, bro. It's all good."

"Thanks, Cody. You're fine now, though, right?" I asked. "Cool. That was pretty damn brave, talking like that. Thank you. Really brave, actually.

"Okay, next, show of hands, who here has had a grandparent with cancer, not passed away necessarily, but was fighting it, kind of like me?"

About half of the class raised a hand.

"Look around, everybody. That's a lot of people. Keep your hands up, okay? Now, how many of you have an aunt or uncle or cousin, same deal as before?"

More hands went up. Over three-quarters of the class now had a hand in the air.

"How about a brother or sister? Or a parent? A really close relative?"

Every hand but one went up in the air. A girl in the front row sat with her arms crossed, face looking down at her desk.

I said, "Look around. Every single one of you has had their life touched by cancer and you guys are freshmen: thirteen, fourteen years old, and already, cancer's a part of your life."

A voice came from the back of the room. "Hey, Mr. S, Bree don't have her hand up. You said everyone had their hand up."

"Indeed. Bree doesn't have her hand up. But remember I said, 'You don't have to play if you don't want to.' And I'm guessing Bree doesn't feel like playing. So yeah, I sort of skipped over her."

Bree looked up at me from the front row with red eyes.

"Hey, Mr. Stanley. It's okay, I mean, I don't want to think about it, and here we're talking about it, but, well, I live with my grandparents. My Mom was having some trouble, okay? And I can't live with my Dad, so I moved in with them. It's cool. They're way out in White Lake, but it's cool, but um, well, Grammy has cancer, and, um…"

"Bree, it's okay, you don't need to say anything, I'm really sorry that you're here for this. If you need…"

"Nah, it's okay. I mean, I feel so fucking useless, oh, sorry about the f-bomb, maybe if I talk about it. Anyway, Grammy is probably gonna die soon, she smokes like a frickin' chimney, and she has cancer of the esophagus. She's had all this surgery, and she has this tube in her stomach 'cause she can't eat, and I take care of her a lot, cause Granpa just can't handle it, I bathe her, and help her in the bathroom, and I gotta take care of food and stuff, so anyway, right around when school started, she got really sick again and the doctors said there wasn't really anything more they could do, so Grammy, well, we're all just kinda waiting for her die, and I just can't, this is such bullshit, and if she goes, maybe I have-ta go back with my Mom, cause Grandpa is just weird about all this, and I just don't know what the Hell to do…"

The red eyes started crying. Quiet cries at first, with Bree's hands at her chest, quickly followed by sobs, and choking sounds, as she tried to hold back. I heard the scrape of Ashlee's chair as she made her way across my classroom. Ashlee wrapped her arms around her friend as Bree sobbed into Ashlee's hair.

"Bree, Ashlee, I want you guys to head down to Ms. Grey in Counseling. I'm calling her right now to tell her whatever she is doing, she needs to drop, and see you right away. Bree, you're a kid, and your being a parent to your grandparents is awesome, but we gotta get you some help at taking care of everybody. Ms. Grey is amazing, and she'll take care of you. Go. Go right now. Thank you, Ashlee, for being such a good friend."

I walked to the door with Ashlee and Bree. I rubbed the back of their necks as they walked out. I watched Bree's head bob as she cried. I watched Ashlee care for her friend. I started welling up.

I walked to the front of classroom. Sniffling with tears, I looked out at my first hour students. Through my own misty eyes, I did not see a dry eye in the dimly lit room.

A voice came from the back of the room. "Yeah, cancer frickin' sucks. Glad you're back, Mr. Stanley."

To Teach What It Means to be a Good Human

It was good to be back in the classroom. A classroom is one of the few places where a public display of raw and powerful emotion like Bree's could become a teachable moment of un-matched intensity. I guarantee that in five, ten, twenty, years, one of the kids in my first hour, now an adult, will be sitting with a friend in need. That kid'll flash back to the kindness shown by Ashlee, or the empathy shown by entire class, or the courage shown by Bree, and will draw forth strength from that moment.

Fortunately, my second and third hour did not have anyone who shared a story as heart-wrenching as Bree's from first hour. We had students who had lost loved ones. We had students who had seen great suffering. But no one else had been subject to the same overwhelming combination, and no one else had been forced so young into such an adult role.

Like their first hour brethren, the kids in second and third hours all complained about Mr. Snape, the substitute teacher. They were glad to have their "real teacher" back. They all gasped when I showed them my scar. They all paid attention to the warning signs of skin cancer, promised to nag their parents, and promised to blame it all on me if their parents didn't like being nagged. As planned, the kids also made fun of my brain on DVD.

By lunch time, I was spent. Exhausted. Done and dusted. Through a fortuitous piece of unplanned schedule-making luck, I was given the first of our three lunch periods, followed by my prep period. Due to the extra passing time required for students to get back and forth from lunch, this gave me an extra 20 minutes of down-time. In short, I had nearly 90 minutes of time in my room without students.

No classroom in our 1,200 student building is as far from the staff lunch room as mine. On a pre-cancerous day, with empty halls, at a brisk pace, the walk would take between three and four minutes. As tired as I was, in halls clogged with loitering and shuffling teens, it would be more like a six-minute slog. Throughout the morning, I had dosed my energy output carefully. Lunch was no exception. As a brown-bagger, I opted to eat at my desk, and save time and energy.

Soup. Yogurt. Salty snack. Fruit. Iced tea.

Nap.

Prior to my surgery, my wife purchased a camp chair for me; complete with head rest, foot rest, arm rest, and cupholder. It sat in the corner of my classroom, wrapped in its own dufflebag. During the first week of school, before my surgery, it was a great place to sit and grade papers during my prep time. Cath's ulterior motive, however, was far more thoughtful. She knew, ahead of my surgery, that I would need a nap to get through the day. She had also purchased several relaxation CDs for me.

Normally, I do not have any difficulties getting to sleep. I read for a few minutes. I take off my glasses and turn out the lights. My head hits the pillow and aside from a 2 am trip to the loo, I sleep. At 5:30 am, my light bulb alarm clock gradually gains brightness as it wakes me, gently, from 8½ hours of sound sleep.

Normally. But it's two weeks post-cancer surgery and "normally" has been tossed in the dumpster. I rarely napped before, and never at school. Until now.

Open up the chair. Turn out the lights. Mute the classroom phone. Sprawl exhaustedly into camp chair. Noise reduction headphones on. Relaxation CD on low. Phone alarm set to vibrate and placed in lap. Listen to 90 seconds of a gentle voice coaxing me over pan flute music to find a "quiet place on a warm beach in my mind."

Next thing I knew, my alarm was vibrating gently on my lap (a treat in itself) to awaken me to face my last classes of the day. It was 40 minutes of heaven. Make some coffee, get my lesson plans together for the next day, and I was ready for my last two classes.

Just as 2nd and 3rd hour went easily, so did 5th and 6th. I packed up, drove the thirty minutes home, and collapsed on the couch for an hour long nap.

No relaxation CD needed; I was in bed by 8:00 pm.

Tuesday dawned another lovely day. A 5:45 am shower. Coffee, oatmeal, a hard-boiled egg, juice, more coffee in the travel mug and I was out the door by 6:40 am. Headed south, Garrison Keillor accompanied me on the CD player with the news from Lake Wobegon. It felt comfortable to be back in the car on I-75 as the sun rose over my left shoulder. I am a creature of habit. Driving to work as the sun rises in September, hanging my polo shirts in Roy G. Biv order in my closet, arranging my CDs alphabetically by artist within musical genre; those

138

are my habits. Those habits make me feel warm and comfortable. Cancer is not a part of my habits.

As I pulled into the teacher's lot, I saw my Science Department chair Lachelle Lemmons as she pulled into her parking space in the conversion van she called "Big Red." For the last six years, with not a femtosecond of planning between us, we'd pulled into the parking lot together at least 80% of the time. Yesterday was one of the 20% days and we had not seen each other.

"Stanley!!" she shrieked.

"LEMMONS!" I yelled back.

We hugged. I accidentally dropped my travel mug. It hit the ground on its bottom edge. Ka-thunk.

My mug bounded up into the air. Still hugging, we looked down, heads swiveling simultaneously, as the mug flipped up into the air, slowly pivoted one hundred and eighty degrees and landed on the edge of the lid. Breaking our grip on each other, we leapt back as the lid popped free from the mug and my coffee sloshed out onto the tarmac.

I bent over, slowly, suddenly conscious of my incipient scar, as I reached under a car to retrieve my mug. Lachelle stood with her arms full, book bags bulging with papers, and her laptop case, and handed me my mug lid as I arose.

"Damn," she said. "Sorry about that coffee. That's no way to start out your second day back."

"If losing some coffee is the worst part of my day, Chelle, then I'll be pretty damn happy at 2:40 when we get out of here," I said.

"Good point," she noted. "Let's go do this. I am so glad to have our Chief Optimism Officer back. You perk people up. You know that, don't you?"

"Um, kind of. I don't know how much is for *their* benefit, and how much is for *mine*, but yeah, being gloomy has never been a thing; I just never saw the sense in being Debbie Downer. Not much fun there. You gotta maximize the fun. So, yeah, let's go teach these kids up, Lemmons. Damn, good to see you, too. Thanks."

As I stood in the doorway to my classroom, fiddling with my keys, I became conscious of the shuffling of feet on the carpet behind me.

"Yeeeessssss?" I said, without turning around.

"Stan-man, can Bree and I talk to you for a minute, kind of in private?"
It was Ashlee.

"Sure. No worries. What's up?"

"Oh, we just need to talk to you for a second. But not out here, okay?"

"Uh, sure. Yeah. Why don't you guys head back into the prep room?

Soon as I get my computer booted up, get the lesson for the day up on the SmartBoard, I'll be right back."

With thirty or forty teachers all trying to log onto the server around the same time, logons are always slow. It was ten minutes before I got everything squared away for the morning. A nervous-looking pair of fourteen-year-old girls were waiting for me. I left the prep room door open. It is a fact of life in modern teaching that one should never be alone with a student, male or female, behind a closed door.

"So, um, Mr. Stanley, Bree has something to say…"

"Ashlee, I can do this… Okay, well, um, anyway, about yesterday…" her voice trailed off.

"Yes?"

"Well, I met with Ms. Grey, she's awesome, just like you said, and she said she's gonna get like Family and Child Services, not Protective Services, you know, but the good guys, to help me out. She's gonna get some nurses out to the house to help with Grammy and stuff like check on my Grandpa, and make sure we have enough food. She's gonna get a caseworker to meet with us cause we prob'ly should get WIC, or food stamps or something, so anyway, things should get lots better and I'm really sorry about crying and dropping that F-bomb and can I hug you?"

"Yeah, I guess we can hug. Guy teachers hugging girls, you know I think that's a little creepy, right? But I guess, since Ashlee's here, okay."

We hugged. I don't have a daughter. It had been a long time since I hugged a teenaged girl. Like since I was a teenaged boy, most likely.

We stepped apart after a few moments.

Bree looked at me and Ashlee.

"Now you."

Ashlee and I looked at each other.

"I'm not hugging him," she said with a smile.

"No way I'm hugging her," I said, smiling back.

"Good God, you two are dense. Not each other, Ash, me. Hug me."

Ashlee and I looked at each other.

"Ohhhhh," we both said.

Today, Tuesday, would be my first day teaching content. But the day before, Monday, I did a boatload of teaching. I suggest that my students will remember Monday's lessons far longer than they would remember today's lesson on the scientific method, but the state mandated tests don't offer a standardized, high stakes test on being a good human.

To teach what it means to be a good human: that is what I missed when I was home.

No Sweat; It's Just Some Dead Skin

The cancer is gone. The cancer story continues. I wish I had a big bang to end my melanoma story, but I don't. My epiphany, like most epiphanies, took a while to grab hold. My life changed in small ways; more compassion, less sarcasm, more heart, tiny changes that created a gradual yet great change. I noticed that I had both gained and lost patience.

For those in need, those who tried, those who struggled, those who put forth honest effort, those of substance, my patience was near limitless. But for those whose concerns were with appearances, with status, with essentially meaningless external identifiers, I now had no patience at all. It was as if I now had two in-baskets. The former basket was immense. The more I put into my "in-basket of heart," the more bottomless it became.

For the "in-basket of conceit," I had nothing. Professor Lawrence Krauss once was asked what would happen if someone fell into a black hole. He replied that you'd be crushed like chunky salsa. That's what happened to issues that fell into my in-basket of conceit.

In short, my life went on. I went back to work. My temporary facelift was, indeed, temporary. The skin on the left side of my face went back to its regular, slightly saggy, 50-year-old self. I continued to nap through a goodly portion of my prep hour. I listened to CDs on healing one's self on my headphones whilst I dozed.

I began to train again. I rode the bike trainer at a walking pace. I gradually increased the load: first in volume, and then in intensity. Once I got the all clear to strain the tissues around my neck, I hit the weight room again. Self-awareness is bad when one trains hard. One needs to be able to dive in, 100% in the moment, to achieve peak performance.

It took a long time to get back to the moment. I had to re-learn how to focus on pain. Every athlete wins because they do not fear pain,

they welcome pain. Pain is where races are won. The first reps are easier, the middle few are more difficult, and the last reps are a deep and
dark hole. You need to welcome that place. But when one wonders if a
six-inch suture line might spring open, or a few wandering melanoma
cells will use the circulatory system as a highway to one's brain, one
goes up to edge of the cliff, teeters a bit, and peers over, rather than
diving right in.

I continued to see Dr. Barkey. Never was I so glad to disrobe before another man as I was in his office. The first six months after my
surgery, I saw him, or more accurately, he saw me, every month. The
second six months, I went in every other month, and for the second
year, we met quarterly. Today, in 2015, mainly at my insistence, we
meet twice a year.

There have been bumps along the way. In 2008, several years after
my surgery, Cath noted a spot on my cheek. My left cheek. Cath didn't
panic. I will say that I have never seen my wife as forceful as she was
that afternoon. She was Lombardi and Ditka rolled into one.

"I don't know what you are planning on doing this afternoon. But
first, you will call Barkey's office and get in there tomorrow. I don't care
if you have to show up at his office at 6:30 am and sit there all day, I am
not going to let you wait around to get this looked at. It is brown, it is
new, and it is on the same side of your face, and now, right now, you
call Barkey's office."

I called.

Barkey keeps a "secret appointment" time for emergencies.

"Be here at 6:30 am. Doctor will see you first thing."

I was there at 6:15 am. I was sitting in the parking lot, doing my
deep breathing, as the office lights came on. Cath may have been Ditka
& Lombardi tough. I was Panic in Detroit scared. At 6:25 am, I was
knocking on the front door. Dr. Walt himself let me in.

"Let's see what we have. C'mon back. You can take care of the paperwork on the way out."

I followed Dr. Barkey down the dark hall into "my" exam room. I
hoisted myself into the chair. He flipped on the exam light at the chair
side and leaned in. Once again, I could feel his breath on my face.
It was calm and regular. I concentrated on my breathing—deep and
slow.

I felt his finger pressing on and around the new brown thing. I
heard him feel around in his pocket for his polarized light source
and magnifier. I heard it click on. Out of the corner of my left eye, I
could feel the intensity of its bright light. He held it there for a few

minutes. I could feel the warmth as he moved it around the area of the lesion.

It snapped off.

"You're fine."

"Whew," escaped quietly from my mouth.

"What is it, then?"

"Ah, some skin thing. You're not gonna make me give you the Greek or Latin, are you? Really, it's nothing. Hang on a sec."

He reached around and took an instrument resembling a dental tool from a counter.

"Hold still."

I heard a scrape. He held the instrument out in front of my face. A small piece of brownish dead skin dangled from its end.

"Just some dead skin. Don't know why it's brown, don't know why it died, but I promise you, it is nothing. Don't worry. It was flaky. It's a rule. 'Don't fear the flake.'

"See you back in six months. You're doing great. The ladies up front will take care of the paperwork on your way out."

I may have skipped and whistled down the hallway to the receptionist's desk. I am certain I frolicked and gamboled. I checked out, gladly forked over the co-pay, and hopped in the car. I had taken the entire day off. If I had received bad news, I knew that work was not the place I'd want to be. I turned the key, turned on the CD player, and the Talking Heads *Once in a Lifetime* blasted at me. Ah, sweet musical synchronicity. I headed north on I-75 at 70 mph; me and the Heads singing *"Letting the days go by, letting the days go by, letting the days go by, once in a lifetime…"*

I walked in the house. Cath was seated on the couch. She sprang up, and before she could say anything, I said, "It's nothing. Just some flaky weird brown skin."

I met her a few steps in front of the couch. We hugged so hard that you couldn't have shoved a dollar bill between us.

"I was so scared," she said. "You've been so good about all of this, and then…"

"You were scared? I was fucking terrified."

"But you never said anything. I didn't know."

"Hell, it wouldn't have done any good, not until we had some data. I figured that if it was good news, then, no big deal. And if it was bad news, then there'd be plenty of time to panic later on. But, scared? Hell yeah, I was scared."

A tear dripped down Cath's face. And then a second, and a third. I felt it on my cheek. A tear dripped down my face. My tear.

WhattheHell, I thought. And another. And another.

We hugged. We swayed. Our tears mingled as they rolled down our cheeks. I was glad I'd taken the day off. There was no place else I needed to be, wanted to be, than sharing hugging space with my wife.

There were also unintended hijinks. In 2010, I went out for a haircut over winter break. I sat in the chair and Sharon, my long-time hair cutter said, "Well, what are we doing today?"

"Oh, I don't know. I've always wondered what I'd look like with a shaved head. Cut it all off."

"Son, you are crazy. You have this beautiful white hair and you want to cut it off? No. Besides, your wife will be in here all in my face and I do not need that."

"Ah, it'll grow back. C'mon. All of it."

"I will, but if your wife shows up, I most definitely do not have your back."

I walked in the door with a shaved head.

"Hey, dear," I said.

"What the hell have you *done*?"

"I've always wanted to see what I looked like with a shaved head."

"Now you know. Don't do that again."

"I won't. Agreed. Once is enough."

Said our 17-year-old son Aaron, "That's so not you, Dad. Not you at all."

My 78-year-old Dad was succinct.

"You look stupid."

Two weeks later, at the conclusion of winter break, I was back at school and the unintended consequences hit home. A few of my colleagues liked it. A few didn't like it. But on Wednesday, two days after school had started, our kindly and quietly snarky administrative assistant Michelle took me aside. The Michelles of the world, as we all know, rule the world.

"Listen, Stanley, I've been asked by a lot of the kids and few of the staff. Are you okay? I mean, you just had cancer a few years ago. I figured you were fine, you were so upfront about your cancer the last time, but people are wondering if it's back. Are you bald from chemo and radiation, or is this just, ahem, a fashion statement? Because if it's a statement, it looks like crap. And if you're sick again, well, people are concerned. So, I thought I'd ask."

I explained my spur of the moment impulse. Michelle gave a deep breath. We hugged.

"Thank God," she whispered.

"Yep," I whispered back. "Thank God. And thank you for asking."

Melanoma: It Started With a Freckle

I went to classroom and sat in front of my PC for a few moments before composing an email to the staff.

Dear friends,

It has been brought to my attention (Thank you, Michelle!) that my newly bald head has caused an unintentional stir. I am fine. Went out for a haircut over break and, God knows why, told my hair cutter to shave my head. Won't do that again—it's too cold in Michigan—I need to wear a hat all the time. At any rate, I was just checked by my cancer specialist a few weeks ago, and I'm fine—no cancer; no chemo or radiation needed. It was nothing but a random "Hey, Look!! A Squirrel!" moment. Please let any kids who ask know that I am fine, and I am truly touched by their concern. Ditto for any of you guys who asked Michelle to ask me. You are the best colleagues anywhere. Thanks. Love you guys.

Cancer, it's a heartless bastard. I got lucky. My wife noticed something. I got to a good doctor early, and he got me the best care possible. The CDC reports that 6,002 men and 3,152 women—9,154 USA citizens—died of melanoma in 2012.

9,154 people dead. More than one per hour.

Dr. Barkey and I discussed this early on in my treatment.

"David, it's a good thing we're taking care of this now. If you'd have waited a year, we'd be talking about an entirely different set of surgical procedures; huge amounts of tissue would be involved, probably some brain surgery, lymph nodes, everything bad about head and neck cancer. And if you'd waited *two years*, there'd be no need to have this conversation. Because you'd be dead."

In December of 2012, I lost my younger brother Michael to squamous cell cancer of his tongue. He was 50. A man who never used tobacco and who rarely drank, Michael lost a terrible roll of the genetic dice. We were both about the same age when skin cancer struck. We both had lesions slightly smaller than a pencil eraser. Mine was in front of my ear. His was on the top of his tongue. Michael also received exceptional and early medical care. For no reason other than sheer random chance, I lost my baby brother.

Six months later, in the summer of 2013, I visited with Dr. Barkey for my semi-annual inspection. (Pro tip: always wear clean underwear to the dermatologist when you are scheduled for your full-body check.) Dr. Barkey had a third-year medical student in tow. Dr. Barkey was well aware that I had just lost my younger brother to a particularly virulent strain of squamous cell cancer of the tongue just several months earlier.

"Dave, I feel the need to remind you that the cancer which took your brother, and the melanoma which you had—neither has a strong genetic component. I mean, you've got a master's, I'm sure you've done the research, but I want you to hear it from me. In your particular case, as long as you continue to practice good sun hygiene, you're no more likely, five or six years post-cancer, to have a recurrence of melanoma than any other guy in the population. Further out from that, it's too soon to tell, but you're good, you'll keep getting checked, right?

"As for your brother's cancer? It was a horrible roll of the dice, he didn't smoke or chew or have a drinking problem, yes? But that's what it was. His kind of squamous cell may have been genetic in the sense that his genes turned those cancer cells loose, you know what I mean here, right? But as far as this being passed onto his kids, or both of you getting it from your parents, that's very unlikely.

"You can stop worrying. I know. Not possible."

"Thanks, I appreciate hearing that," I said. "That's exactly what I read in the literature, but hearing it from you, I know you stay current, makes me feel better. And yes, you will be seeing me. Regularly. I promise."

"If it's okay with you, I'm going to do your full exam, and then my student will take a look at your face and arms, we'll hear from him, and then I'll tell him what he saw correctly, and what he may have missed."

I removed my shoes and socks. I dropped my pants.

Barkey started out between my toes, up my legs, behind my knees, the fronts of my thighs. He pulled out the waistband of my drawers. I pushed my willy first to one side, then the other, as he inspected my groin. I raised my penis and scrotum while he peered at my perineum. I turned and he inspected the space between my buttocks.

"Um-hmm. Good," he murmured.

I removed my shirt.

Barkey scoured my torso and upper limbs: front and back, under my arms, down my arms to my hands, between the fingers, under the fingernails. He pointed out a meaningless skin tag to his student. He showed him the difference between a small mole and a freckle. He peeked under my tongue and the inside of my cheeks. He did his usual ultra-careful inspection of my face and neck: behind the ears, parting the hairs on my neck, in the corners of my eyelids, everywhere he knew melanoma to strike.

He turned to his student.

"Your patient."

The young man mimicked Dr. Barkey's paths over my chest and back. I could hear him breathing. He was not calm. As he spotted freckles, small moles, and skin tags, he announced them aloud in a nervous voice. As he inspected my chest, and under my arms, small beads of sweat were visible on his forehead. Understandable. Here he was doing an exam in front of the chief, with a patient who read medical journals in his spare time.

As he worked his way down to my hands, I could feel his rapid pulse as it thumped in his thumbs when he held my arm up for inspection. He took a long look at a bright pink, half-dollar sized blemish between my right thumb and forefinger.

"Dr. Barkey, what about this?"

He held my hand out for inspection.

"Should we be concerned about this?"

Barkey looked at me and raised an eyebrow.

"You want to tell him about that, Mr. Stanley?"

"Sure thing."

I turned to the young man.

"I burned the crap out of my hand on the grill a few weeks ago. Second degree. Smelled just like chicken."

Barkey walked over to the young man and patted him on the back. "You did well."

He smiled at the still-nervous young man.

"You weren't sure what that burn thing was. I knew. Good that you got your question answered. Nice work."

Barkey turned back to me.

"Look, you've been clean ever since your surgery. There's really no reason for you to come back again, unless your wife spots something. You are in the perfect place, you know. A wife who knows what to look for, and loves you enough to look.

"I can set you free with no qualms on my part."

I must have looked either disappointed, or alarmed.

"Right. I get it. I'll humor you. You're good company around the office. See you in January."

Nearly Dying is a Blessing

Small things matter.

Thanks to small things, I am alive. First of all, my wife loves me. She likes to stroke the bridge of my nose—yes, like a puppy. Whilst stroking my nose, she happened to notice that "weird looking freckly thing" just in front of my left ear's tragus. It was small—as small as a peppercorn. But to her R.N., B.S.N., M.S.N.-trained mind, it just didn't look right. At that moment, as Dr. Barkey said on several occasions, my melanoma was an easy fix. In one year, it's a much more drastic set of procedures. In two years, there are no procedures.

Because I'm dead.

Small things. Cath loved my nose. She looked at me. I write these words. She doesn't love to touch my face…

Sun feels good. Use it carefully.

As a young man, I spent too much time, unprotected time, in the sun. Sun feels great on your skin. From childhood to young adulthood, I played tennis and soccer all summer long. I loved how it looked. I loved how it felt. It felt healthy. It felt sexy.

No sun screen required.

In my twenties, as a semi-pro traveling bicycle racer, I can't forget that I spent two to five hours each day, nearly seven days each week, from February and March (in Texas) through to September on a bike saddle. Twenty hours of pure UV each week, for thirty-two weeks every year. Nearly all of it unprotected.

Stupid.

When you work in the yard, slap on sunscreen and a hat. When you head out to golf course, or for a bike ride, glop on some lotion. It's such a cheap, easy and effective fix. Because most of us use far too little sunscreen, an SPF below 30 is too low to be effective. Above 50, any increase in sun protection is negligible, although the costs are not. It takes about one ounce, a shot glass worth, of sunscreen to adequately cover arms, legs, head, and neck.

Nearly dying is a blessing.

Nearly dying is a blessing. Many of us have re-invented ourselves: new school, new job, new neighborhood; but only those of us who have seriously looked at death have had the blessing of almost dying.

It's not the pain and suffering. Quite frankly, pain and suffering are wildly over-rated as a means to attain enlightenment; ghostly white monks in *The Da Vinci Code* notwithstanding. Many of us have endured a lot of crap in the name of medical science. But it is not pain that is the blessing. It is the opportunity to truly see one's own demise, not merely to contemplate one's death (said staring at skull in hand, "alas, poor David"), and return to the living with love and vigor.

My father Mort, a retired physician, did it. He did it well. As a younger man, I am told, Mort suffered fools far less gladly than most. Loudly and angrily was how he suffered them. He was a hard-charger, the Dad, as were many men and women who grew up during the Depression.

If you didn't bust ass, you didn't eat.

Dad smoked. A lot.

Dad guzzled coffee. A lot.

Dad worked his butt off, long after he needed to. In 1992, it caught up with him. A sore calf led to a diagnosis of claudication which led to a diagnosis of severe blockages of a variety of coronary arteries which led to multiple coronary artery bypasses which led to a then 62-year-old man reaching his 84th (and counting, as of 2015) birthday.

Somewhere between Friday's marching orders of "Mort, go home, put your feet up. DO NOT MOVE. We're doing you on Monday" and Monday, Mort realized that (as the kids say) "Shit about to get real."

A quick story about Mort in pre-op on that Monday morning. There is Dad laying on the gurney, Lois, the Mom, at his side. The anesthesiologist strolls over.

"Mort, you know the drill. Blah blah blah blah blah. Oh, are you a smoker?"

"No," says Mort.

Lois belts him so hard on the shoulder that the gurney rattled.

"I'm not," he protests. "I quit on Friday."

Epiphany found its way to Mort. Epiphany liked Mort plenty. It liked Mort so much that it took up permanent residence in his born-again heart. He learned that working 16 hours per week in the Family Practice Clinic training new docs was pretty darn satisfying. He learned that food tasted a lot better when not filtered through tar and nicotine. He found that the aromatic in gin was juniper, not tobacco. He found that one can get stuff done without losing one's temper. And vacations could really last longer than four days.

It was the blessing of almost dying. Mort sprinted right up to the edge of the abyss and peeked over, teetered there for a few moments, and decided that changing paths was a whole lot wiser than charging down one that was a guaranteed dead end.

It happens to everyone who looks quite seriously at death. My realization first came when Dr. Barkey called at 7:00 pm on a Thursday evening and said, "You need to be at my office first thing tomorrow so we can discuss your treatment options."

It happened to me again, in the summer of 2013. My pulled rib muscle was instead a massive pulmonary embolism, so large that I was confined to bed until the medications went to work, so concerned was the care team that walking to the loo might break a chunk of clot loose, whence it might lodge in my heart and kill me.

No more bad days. I now lead a charmed life.

Many people have far more moving and painful stories: massive amounts of tissue removed, horribly debilitating radiation and chemo, months and months of rehab to re-learn basic movements and skills.

But we all did the same thing. We got shoved and steamrollered right up to the edge, and somehow, we didn't fall into the crevasse. When we came back, we were different. Not superficially different—made-over and lost weight and new wardrobe different—but wholly changed in a fundamental way.

We got it, right down to our soul. Every day matters. Every freakin' day. Each time you awake, you matter. To yourself, your loved ones, to the world.

The lessons cancer taught me:
- You may think, "Hey wait a sec, I did not sign up for this." Sorry, bro. Tag. You're it.
- Few of us realize our legacy whilst still alive. Here's your chance. Grab onto it. Fiercely. Create that legacy.
- Find peace and contentment in ways that were not open to you before. Smell the flowers. Compliment the stranger. Pray, meditate, contemplate.
- Be a source of strength and inspiration to those you meet. Allow others to inspire you. Draw strength from those who care about you.
- Accept the blessing of nearly dying.
- Merely by being the best you can be, you are blessed every day.

The Three Faces of Skin Cancer

Basal Cell Carcinoma:

Basal cell carcinoma (BCC) begins in the basal cells of the skin. This layer is responsible for the production of new skin cells as old cells die. BCCs typically resemble open sores. They can also looks like small, waxy bumps, red patches, or scars. They rarely metastasize (spread) beyond the original location. It is even more rare that they become life-threatening. However, they can be become quite disfiguring if left untreated. BCCs are generally caused by long-term exposure to UV radiation caused by sunlight.

Squamous Cell Carcinoma:

Squamous cell carcinoma (SCC) arises in the squamous cells of the skin. These cells comprise most of the skin's uppermost layer, the epidermis. Squamous means "scale-like." An SCC can take many shapes: a scaly red patch, a wart, or an open sore. They often appear as raised growths with a low spot in the middle, as if it were a very small volcanic caldera. They may also crust over and/or bleed. While SCCs can disfigure, they can also kill. Six to eight thousand people die annually from squamous cell cancer.

While most SCCs are a result of sun damage, SCCs may occur on anywhere on the body. This includes mucus membranes, genitalia, and those areas typically exposed to the sun. A squamous cell lesion, about the size of a pencil eraser, on my brother's tongue took his life in December of 2012.

Melanoma:

Melanoma is cancer of the melanocytes. The melanocytes are the pigment cells within the skin. Melanoma is the most serious form of skin cancer. Any place where pigment cells can be found can give rise to melanoma. This includes the eye, and rarely, the membranes of the nose, mouth, and pharynx, as well as the vaginal and anal mucosa.

However, most pigment cells are found in the skin, and this is where most melanomas are found. Around 70% of all melanomas begin in or near an existing mole or dark spot on the skin. This is why it is important to visit your health care provider any time a mole appears to have grown, changed, or in some way, "looks different." Most melanomas, around 90%, are associated with UV exposure via sunlight.

However, one specific type of melanoma—acral lentiginous melanoma—is not closely correlated with sun damage. This cancer is the most common subtype amongst Asian and black individuals. It is found on non-hairy surfaces: the palms, soles, under the nails, and in the oral mucosa.

The ABCs of Skin Cancer

A is for ASYMMETRY.

Draw a line through the middle of your mole. Do the two sides present mirror images? That means they are symmetrical. If the two sides do not match up, they are *asymmetrical* and you need to see your health care provider.

B is for BORDER.

In a benign mole, the edges, like a bean, are smooth and even. In a potentially malignant lesion, the edges are often scalloped, erose, or saw-toothed.

C is for COLOR.

Most benign moles are one color. Most often, they are a single shade of brown or beige. A mole of several colors, or of several shades of the same color, should raise a warning flag and you need to see your health care provider.

D is for DIAMETER.

Benign moles are usually smaller in diameter than malignant moles. Most melanomas are bigger than ¼ inch. But not always. Watch it. Because...

E is for EVOLVING.

Any changes in a mole or spot on the skin need to be investigated. All changes—size, color, shape, height—need to be examined. Any new symptom—bleeding, itching, discharge, or crusting—is likewise a danger signal.

Appendix III
Skin Cancer by the Numbers

In general:

1. Twenty percent of Americans, over their lifetimes, will have skin cancer.
2. Every year, 5 million people in the US are treated for skin cancer. BCC is the most common form. Around 3 million people are diagnosed annually. SCC is the second most common. Around 700,000 people are diagnosed every year.
3. Since 1985, more people have had skin cancer than all other cancers combined.
4. If you live to be 65, the odds are 1 in 2 that you will have at least one basal cell or squamous cell carcinoma.
5. Organ transplant patients are up to 250 times more likely than the general public to develop SCC.
6. Actinic keratosis (AK), a rough and scaly patch that develops after years of UV exposure, is the most common pre-cancer. These affect nearly 60 million Americans.
7. About 65% of SCCs and 35% of BCCs arise in lesions that were previously noted as AKs.

Melanoma:

1. One person dies every hour from melanoma.
2. About 75,000 new cases of melanoma will be diagnosed in 2015.
3. There are about 1,000,000 people alive today with a history of melanoma.
4. In the early 1950s, you had a 50/50 chance of dying if you were diagnosed with melanoma. Today, the odds are better than nine out of ten that you will survive.
5. Melanoma is a growing danger:
   - Of the seven most common cancers in the US, melanoma is the only one whose incidence is growing.

- Melanoma, along with esophageal and liver cancers, are the only cancers with an increasing mortality rate for men.
- Melanoma survivors are NINE times more likely to develop a new melanoma.
- Melanoma is the most common form of cancer amongst those age 25–29.

6. Sun and UV exposure are the key dangers:
    - Nine out ten melanomas are related to UV exposure.
    - The vast majority of DNA mutations in melanoma are UV related.
    - Five or more sunburns as a youth increases melanoma risk by 80% as an adult.
    - Regular use of SPF 15, or greater, sunscreen cuts your risk of melanoma in half.

7. Early detection and treatment are paramount:
    - When treated before the tumor has spread to the lymph nodes, the survival rate is 98%.
    - Once the disease reaches the lymph nodes, the survival rate drops to 63%.
    - Once metastasized to distant organs, survival rates fall to 16%.

Men vs. Women

1. The death rate from melanoma is 65% male, 35% female.
2. From 1970 to 2004, melanoma has more than doubled amongst women and increased 60% amongst men.
3. Women 39 and under have a greater chance of developing melanoma than any cancer except breast cancer.
4. The majority of melanoma diagnoses are white men over 50.

Tanning is evil

1. Ultraviolet radiation is a carcinogen. The WHO includes UV radiation on their Group 1 list of the world's most dangerous carcinogens. This list includes plutonium, cigarettes, benzene, X-rays, and gamma radiation.
2. More people develop skin cancer from tanning than get lung cancer from smoking.
3. Nearly 500,000 cases of skin cancer are linked to indoor tanning.
4. UV damage from tanning is cumulative:
    - One indoor tanning session increase the risk of SCCs by 67%.
    - Six tanning sessions as a teen increases the risk of BCCs by 75%.
    - Sixty seconds in the average tanning machine is twice as carcinogenic as one minute in the noon day sun in the deserts of North Africa.

5. Do not believe the tanning industry hype. There is no such thing as a "safe" tanning machine. The indoor tanning industry generates five billion dollars annually.

Skin cancer strikes all ethnicities

1. Melanoma is rare amongst people of color; 1 per 100,000 in blacks, 4 per 100,000 in Hispanics, and 25 per 100,000 in non-Hispanic whites. However, it is more often fatal. The 5 year survival rate is only 75% in African-Americans vs. 93% for whites.
2. SCC is the most common skin cancer amongst African-Americans and Asian Indians.
3. SCCs in African-Americans are more aggressive. There is a 20-40% chance of metastasis.
4. Melanomas in people of color most often occur on non-exposed skin with less pigment: palms, soles, mucous membranes, and nail regions. (See Appendix I: *Faces of Skin Cancer: Melanoma; acral lentiginous melanoma*)
5. Melanoma is too often a late-stage diagnosis in people of color: 52% for people of color vs 16% in whites.

Skin Aging

1. Over 90% of visible age-related changes are directly related to UV exposure.
2. Regular sunscreen use can lower these changes by 25%.
3. It is a myth that 75% of person's lifetime sun exposure is acquired by 18. Merely 25% of one's lifetime exposure happens as a teen.

The Costs: Follow the Money

1. We spent over $8 billion in 2012 to treat skin cancers:
   - Non-melanoma cancers = $4.8 billion
   - Melanomas = $3.3 billion
2. Since 2002, the costs to treat skin cancers have quadrupled compared to all other cancers.
3. The US economy loses about $3 billion annually in productivity due to melanoma alone.

The statistics quoted above, and in this book, are drawn from fact sheets via the Skin Cancer Foundation, the American Cancer Society, the Mayo Clinic, and the Melanoma Research Foundation websites. In some instances, percentages were rounded for clarity. The statistics are believed to be accurate, but not guaranteed.

About the Author

David L. Stanley, B.Sc., M.A., holds degrees in zoology and teaching. A lifelong athlete, teacher, coach, and freelance writer, his work first appeared in the late, lamented *Bicycle Guide* magazine in 1986. He won the *Peloton/Giordana* writing award in April 2013 for his piece "What Makes a Classic."

Stanley speaks widely on a variety of subjects; among them fatherhood, cancer advocacy, and education. On Twitter, @dstan58 tweets early and often.

The son of a physician, he has had a long time love affair with science and medicine.

He lives in Michigan with his wife and dogs.

www.ingramcontent.com/pod-product-compliance
Lightning Source LLC
Chambersburg PA
CBHW021112090426
42738CB00006B/606